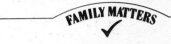

FAMILY MATTERS
✓

A-Z
OF CHILDHOOD
ILLNESSES

DEDICATION

In writing this book I have been able to recall many days and nights when I worried over my own children. My fears were often groundless, but there were times when my concerns as a mother led me to question some of the advice that I was given by the medical profession. All parents should follow their intuition and if you think your child is ill, seek help and don't give up until you get it.

FAMILY MATTERS

✓

A-Z
OF CHILDHOOD
ILLNESSES

ROS MEEK

WARD LOCK

A WARD LOCK BOOK

First published in the UK 1991
by Ward Lock
(a Cassell imprint)
Villiers House
41/47 Strand
LONDON
WC2N 5JE

Distributed in the United States
by Sterling Publishing Co., Inc.
387 Park Avenue South, New York, NY 10016–8810

Distributed in Australia
by Capricorn Link (Australia) Pty Ltd
P.O. Box 665, Lane Cove, NSW 2066

British Library Cataloguing in Publication Data
Meek, Ros
    A–Z of childhood illnesses.
    1. Children. Diseases
    I. Title   II. Series
    618.92

ISBN 0–7063–6969–6

Typeset by Columns Design and Production Services Ltd., Reading

Printed and bound in Great Britain by William Collins & Sons,
Glasgow

CONTENTS

HOW TO USE THIS BOOK

This book is not meant to take the place of a doctor or health professional. It is intended to be a source of basic information about most of the common childhood illnesses.

The first chapters look at the general care of an ill child, first aid and useful things to keep to hand in case of illness. Immunisation, because of its importance as a prevention against disease, has a chapter of its own. The common illnesses are then divided up into sections according to the origin of the illness eg constipation is under Digestive System. I have also included a list of useful organisations where you may be able to get further advice and support.

Don't forget to look after yourself too! Illness occurs when your resistance is lowered by lack of sleep, inadequate diet and stress. If you have been looking after an ill baby, ask your partner to help out with some shopping or cleaning, so that you get a chance to unwind.

Chapter 1

INTRODUCTION

The 20th century has seen great improvements in the health and well-being of the general public. This has resulted in greater life expectancy and an increasing awareness of the need for public health measures that will benefit us all. We take for granted good clean water, sewage waste disposal and measures that seek to prevent industry from polluting the air and rivers.

Amazing discoveries in the medical field have made us feel that there should be a cure for everything, we are able to buy an increasingly wide range of medicines over the counter, and we expect that the medical profession will be able to diagnose and treat most of our illnesses.

The knowledge of how a good diet can affect our health, the encouragement to exercise, stop smoking and restrict alcohol intake, gives us all the opportunity to do something positive to safeguard our families' health.

Once you become a parent for the first time, all these issues take on a greater significance. Good health in pregnancy combined with the antenatal care that is offered, increase the likelihood of a healthy baby. Breastfeeding is one of the best ways of providing a child with some protection against infection in the first few months of its life. By taking advantage of the services of the local child health clinic for immunisation, developmental assessments and advice, your baby will be screened for any abnormalities that might cause a problem in the future. It is the development of these services that has caused the dramatic decline in infectious diseases that used to kill about six in every ten babies in the 1890s.

The measures that have been taken by past governments and local authorities to provide us with this high standard of public health cannot be taken for granted. New diseases such as AIDS and the increasing rates of heart disease, smoking and drug abuse are all matters for public and individual concern. We can help our families by eating and drinking sensibly and setting safe standards of hygiene in our homes.

Despite all the positives about our health these days, we still fall ill, and this can be a great worry when that illness occurs to a baby or child. Illness arrives quickly in most children, one moment they are happily playing and the next they may have a high temperature and be not themselves at all. As a parent you are in an important position. You are the best judge of your baby's health or otherwise; after all, you look after the child most of the time and know how he behaves normally. It therefore follows that if you are concerned about your child's health, you are probably right to be asking for advice. No one likes to feel that they are wasting the time of their GP or health visitor, but these health professionals are used to seeing babies and children, and will quickly reassure you if all is well, or refer you for further help if that is needed. Don't keep your worries to yourself, talk them over with your partner or friend if you want to, but do seek the help of someone who can put your anxieties into perspective.

Chapter 2

THE ILL CHILD AND WHEN TO CALL THE DOCTOR

Parents' anxiety over the health of their child is very natural. Small babies cannot tell you what the problem is and the resultant crying can be extremely distressing for new parents. You may be aware that they are in pain but do not know whether it is in the tummy or lower down. Children get sick faster than adults — one minute they are fine and the next they are drooping and out of sorts perhaps with a high temperature. So how do you tell when it is important to call the doctor?

The most important guide is yourself. You know your child best. You care for him day and night and so you know when he is not behaving normally. If you are worried then that should be enough. Call the doctor and do not be put off if you feel it is urgent. A child with a high temperature or one that you feel is infectious should not be seen in the surgery. If your own doctor is unable to come, then take your child to the nearest casualty department explaining that you have contacted your own GP.

A baby or child needs urgent treatment if there is:

* Severe bleeding
* Severe pain
* Severe burns
* Severe diarrhoea and vomiting — particularly in babies.

☆ Severe blow on the head
☆ Poison or object swallowed (eg safety pin)
☆ A fit or convulsion
☆ Difficulty in breathing
☆ Any unusual and obvious lumps or swellings
☆ You are really worried

Try to think back over the past 24 hours and consider the following list which is particularly relevant to babies.

1. FEEDING DURING THE LAST 24 HOURS

Has your baby/child had its usual amount to drink? An ill child may want to drink more water and juice than the usual amount of milk. The change is most significant if the child is not eating.

If you are breast feeding think about the length of time the baby has fed for and whether he has sucked as strongly as usual. If he has drunk half the amount that he usually takes you should be concerned.

2. VOMITING

Small amounts of posset or milk coming back after a feed are normal. If your baby has a large amount after the last three feeds then you should be concerned. If your baby has vomited a green fluid it means that the vomiting is coming from below the stomach and again is a cause for concern.

3. URINE

Obviously if your child is drinking less and has vomited the number of wet nappies will be less. There can be other reasons though for a child not going to the toilet as often as usual.

4. BLOOD IN THE STOOLS

Large amounts of blood either fresh (red) or black may be seen in the baby or child's bowel motion. It may be a sign of inflammation of the bowel or a blockage. This is a cause for concern.

5. BEHAVIOUR

Ill babies and children become drowsy and less responsive. Is your baby more irritable than usual? Have you had to wake him for a couple of feeds? Is he more fretful or just drowsy all the time? This is important information which will help the doctor to decide what is wrong with your baby. Your baby's cry can also be an indication of illness. Perhaps the cry sounds weak and feeble or high pitched.

The following signs are also important, should be noted and reported to your doctor when you call.

TEMPERATURE

A baby's normal temperature is 37.5°C (98.4°F). It is usually higher if the temperature is taken in the rectum and lower if it is taken under the arm. If the temperature is above 38.3°C (101°F) it is another important sign to tell the doctor. A high temperature on its own does not necessarily mean that the child is ill, it needs to be considered together with the other signs.

RASH

Most babies have a few spots but look for a rash that is more unusual and covers a large area of the body. If the rash is sore and weeping it is also a sign of ill health particularly if larger than 3 cm (1¼ in) square.

SKIN COLOUR

You are the best judge of your baby's normal skin colour. Unusual pallor is an important sign to mention to the doctor.

RESPONSIVENESS

A healthy baby will be alert and according to his age will respond to things around him. Consider if your baby feels more floppy than usual. Perhaps his head is lolling to one side or he is reluctant to move his head. Is he responding to things he normally enjoys and above all is he still interested in you?

BREATHING

A healthy baby breathes very shallowly. In fact it is sometimes hard to tell as all mothers know when they are checking their baby while they sleep. A baby that is ill may suck in the chest or upper part of the tummy. This is an important sign to tell the doctor when you telephone. If your baby is wheezing as he breathes out it is important to tell the doctor.

BUMPS AND BULGES

Look at the baby's groin or scrotum. If there is a bulge that gets larger when the baby cries and disappears when he sleeps, it is most probably a hernia. Hernias in girls are quite rare. Your doctor should see the hernia when it first appears so that he can advise about treatment and possible complications. See page 95.

CIRCULATION

Usually if you squeeze your baby's big toes for a couple of seconds it will make a pale patch. The colour will quickly return when you let go. If the colour does not return to normal within three seconds it means that the baby's circulation of blood is slower than usual. If the fingers or toes appear blue it is also worth mentioning to the doctor.

The above signs should be considered together to help you make up your mind how ill your baby is. No one likes to bother the doctor, but it is important that you get help when you feel it is needed.

SHOCK

Shock can be seen in a child who has had a bad fright, or from a more severe cause such as failure of the circulation and breathing following a bad accident. The child may be shaky and pale, and if the shock involves trauma – such as bleeding or pain – the reaction may be more severe.

What to do

1. Lie the child down so that the head is lower than the feet, thereby aiding the blood flow to the brain.
2. Take care breathing is not obstructed by any vomiting.
3. Keep the child warm but loosen any tight clothing.
4. Reassure and talk to the child.
5. If the child is not better within half an hour, call a doctor.

Severe shock

This needs urgent medical attention. While waiting for help go through the procedure just mentioned but also look for bleeding and stop it.

Chapter 3

LOOKING AFTER AN ILL CHILD

There are very few illnesses that require that a child stays in bed in order to recover. If the child wants to go to bed then let that be your guide, he will want to get up as soon as he feels better. Ill children want company, so often making a child comfortable on the sofa or in the kitchen is better for you both. He will feel less bored and less neglected if he keeps seeing you and it is easier for you to care for him. If the child is being looked after in bed:

* He needs to be kept comfortable. Perhaps a few extra pillows to prop him up. The bed straightened up several times during the day and the bed clothes changed regularly particularly if he has a high temperature and is sweating.
* Keep the room warm and well ventilated. As long as he is not in a draught the window can be opened. Do not overheat the room or it will become stuffy.
* Freshen up. Washing his face and hands will make him feel better. Freshen his mouth with a mouthwash if you cannot get him to clean his teeth. Wash his hands before eating and after using the toilet. Baths are not necessary unless he is very sweaty.
* Boredom is the biggest enemy with ill children. They are away from their friends and their usual activites. Remember that when a child is ill he does not want to

have to try too hard. Choose jigsaws and games that he can do easily.

☆ It is a good idea to keep a few things in a drawer for just such moments. Little felt finger puppets, a few books, a notebook and felt tip pens are all useful.

☆ Cassette tapes are a real boon to an ill child. There are so many available now. Many libraries also have a loan scheme for tapes, so make use of them. Ask other friends too so that you can get a selection that does not drive you mad as you hear the story for the tenth time! Head phones can be used unless the child has an earache or headache which may make it worse. Stories will often lull children off to sleep too!

WHAT TO DO IF YOUR CHILD HAS A FEVER

Children can become feverish very quickly and the temptation is to wrap them up and keep them warm — DON'T. Instead:

1. Take the temperature.
2. Look at the child — he may appear flushed about the face and ears.
3. Remove clothing and some bed clothes. Check the room temperature. The ideal is 20°C (68°F).
4. Give him plenty of drinks and some paracetamol. Read the dosage carefully.
5. If he is very sweaty give him a cool bath. If his temperature is over 39.4° (103°F) he may be too ill to have a bath.

Tepid sponging can have a remarkably quick effect on his temperature.

HOW TO GIVE TEPID SPONGE TREATMENT

1. Protect the bed with a plastic or rubber sheet or towels.
2. Prepare a bowl of warm water and a sponge or flannel.
3. Undress the child and sponge him all over.
4. Do not dry him as the evaporation of water will also help to keep him cool.
5. Leave a cool flannel on his neck and under his arms or groin. Refresh them regularly.
6. Check his temperature about every 10 minutes until it has come down to 37.8°C (100°F).

A fever strip thermometer is very useful to have when tepid sponging.

If you are unable to control the temperature then you may decide to call the doctor. Make a note of the temperature of the child over the past few hours so that the doctor knows the pattern.

A high temperature that is untreated can dehydrate a baby or child and the overheating can lead to a convulsion. A convulsion is a series of muscular spasms which follow a headache or fever. Febrile convulsions tend to recur and so doctors sometimes prescribe anticonvulsant medicine to prevent it happening again.

FEEDING AN ILL CHILD

Many children want nothing to eat when they are ill. Encourage them to drink instead to avoid them becoming dehydrated. You can offer diluted fruit juice, squash or plain water. Milk is often refused. As he starts to accept food offer him a little of whatever he fancies. Do not put large amounts on the plate, he can always ask for more. Small pieces of fruit such as orange segments can tempt a flagging appetite and will also help prevent constipation which often occurs after an illness.

GIVING MEDICINE

Children either like or loathe having medicine and both can cause problems. The child may use his illness to have time off school having seen how mum responds when he is ill. Try not to suggest symptoms to your child as he may exaggerate or invent them later. If you have difficulty giving your baby or child medicine a dropper or syringe may help. There are also special medicine spoons which stop the medicine being spilt if the child is wriggling away!

When the doctor comes and prescribes medicine tell him if the child suffers from any allergies or has had side effects from taking medicine. Make sure that any medicine you give is within the expiry date, and follow the instructions on the bottle. Do not give an extra spoonful as this can be dangerous and use the correct type of medicine spoon. If the child vomits within an hour of taking the medicine give another dose, and do not give a sleeping or sleepy child medicine as he may choke on it.

See page 74 for giving ear drops.
See page 82 for giving eye drops.

GOING INTO HOSPITAL

If your doctor feels that your child needs hospital treatment it can come as a shock to both you and the child. It helps if you can talk about hospitals, doctors and nurses when he is well. Tell him about other children that may have been into hospital, perhaps you have a friend who works in a hospital, all these things will encourage a positive attitude.

Hospital wards are much more welcoming today, but that is not to say that everything will go as you wish. NAWCH, the National Association for the Welfare of Children in Hospital (see page 124) can be very helpful if you have a problem. Talk to your health visitor or GP about what services the hospital can provide i.e. can you stay there, will they provide meals, is there open visiting etc.

WHAT TO TAKE INTO HOSPITAL

Nightie or pyjamas
Dressing gown and slippers
Washing things
Favourite toy or cuddly thing

Do not forget to take the same sort of things in for yourself.

YOU WILL NEED

A change of clothes
A nightie
Washing things
Book or magazine
Change or card for the telephone

It may be very difficult for you to arrange things so that you can be with your child. Children who have regular contact with their parents do tend to have a shorter stay in hospital, so be there as much as you can. Ask friends and neighbours to send a card or postcard — it will cheer him up to know about what others are doing and that they have not forgotten him. If you have financial difficulties ask to see the hospital social worker.

Little things mean a lot to a child in hospital. If you are delayed in visiting, telephone so that the staff can tell your child so that he is not so upset as visitors arrive for other children. Tell the staff if he has particular likes or dislikes, particularly if he sleeps with a light on in the bedroom, is eneuretic (wets the bed) or is on any medication. Ask for information about your child. When you are concerned you do not always take in all the information you may have been given. Ask again or ask for your husband or partner or a friend to be with you.

There are many self-help groups who support parents whose child may have a long term illness or handicap. See pages 122–5 for details.

When your child gets better or comes home from hospital be ready for difficulties. Things that you may have allowed in hospital may turn into habits that you do not want to stay. Be firm but patient. He may start to wet the bed, prefer to be fed or be difficult or negative. This type of rejection is very hard for parents who may feel that now the child is better all will return to normal. It is hard not to spoil a child who has been into hospital, but brothers and sisters will become very jealous if you are over indulgent. Talk about the hospital stay so that any fears can be discussed and allayed in case a further visit to outpatients or to the ward is needed. If your child has to have any special tests performed, talk to your health visitor. She is a qualified nurse and will be able to answer your questions and concerns.

Chapter 4

FIRST AID AND THE MEDICINE CHEST

From the moment that you bring your baby home from the hospital, you will begin to amass creams, ointments and powders all intended to deal with everyday baby care and ailments. Before you leave them on a convenient chest of drawers or on the bathroom shelf it is worth considering the safety aspects of keeping medicines and such products in the home. Although your baby may well be small and helpless now, by one year he will be trying to stand up, crawl and maybe walk. This new-found mobility puts him at risk from falls, knocks and cuts and from the many other possibly dangerous things around the home which we as adults regard as safe.

That little group of previously safe medicines and ointments may well be reachable if he stands on a chair or pushes up a stool to the dressing table. So from the start *before* an accident occurs, keep medicines in a locked cabinet or a cupboard with a cupboard lock (available from all good hardware shops). Tell child-minders, visitors to the house and babysitters where your first aid kit is so that in an emergency it can be found easily. Keep a note of your doctor's telephone number on the door or lid of the box so that it is to hand if necessary.

FIRST AID BOX CONTENTS

Packet of assorted sticking plasters
Roll of sticking plaster for larger cuts
Packet of sterile gauze
Zinc oxide plaster for attaching gauze
Pair of scissors and tweezers
Cotton wool
Crêpe bandage for sprains
Gauze bandage to keep dressing on
Triangular bandage for a sling
A clean fresh handkerchief in a paper bag (to cover a
    larger wound, eg a burn, on the way to hospital)
A thermometer
Safety pins
Eye bath and lotion and eye pad, optional
Pre-packed burns dressing, optional
Butterfly plasters for finger and knuckle injuries

THE MEDICINE CHEST

Paracetamol suspension for infants over 4 months
    tablets for children
5 ml plastic spoon
5 ml plastic syringe (ask your doctor for one if you have
    difficulty getting your child to take medicine)
Calamine lotion for rashes and bites
Insect sting reliever spray
Witch hazel for all kinds of cuts, bruises and bites
Antiseptic lotion to clean cuts and grazes
Antiseptic cream for reddened or infected cuts
Cream for burns such as aloe vera
Nappy rash cream
Multivitamin drops
Vapour chest rub or inhalant capsules for colds
Vaporiser for children prone to chestiness, optional
Plaster mark remover, optional

CAUTION

* ☆ Always ask your doctor or pharmacist if liquid medicine should be kept in the fridge.
* ☆ Some medicines should be taken on an empty stomach. Check with the pharmacist.
* ☆ Always finish the full course of treatment or your child may need a second course.
* ☆ Dispose of old pills and medicines safely. (Ask your pharmacist).
* ☆ Laxatives should not be necessary for babies and children.
* ☆ Eye drops and nose drops should be thrown away once the ailment is cured.
* ☆ If you suspect your child has an allergy or reaction to the medicine, telephone your doctor or pharmacist before discontinuing the course.
* ☆ Keep all of your iron and vitamin pills, contraceptives and other medications locked away too. They can be lethal in large doses.
* ☆ Remember to be alert when you visit relatives or friends — they may not lock away their medicines and tablets.

A–Z OF FIRST AID

BITES AND STINGS

If you are going abroad it is wise to find out about any particular hazards that there might be for yourself and your children. These may range from mosquitoes and snakes in some countries to the fear of rabies.

If your child is bitten or stung by an insect or animal

they will need plenty of reassurance. That a previously friendly dog or horse has turned on them and attacked them is very difficult for a child to understand. Reassurance is therefore his first need.

Most bites need little attention.

☆ Wash the area and dry it. Cover it with a plaster or dry dressing.
☆ Keep an eye on it for signs of infection — redness around the edge of the wound.
☆ Severe bites or punctures to the skin should be seen by a doctor as tetanus injections may be needed or treatment against possible infection.
☆ Snake bites need prompt action.
☆ Reassure the child and treat for shock if necessary.
☆ Lie him down to slow the spread of the poison.
☆ Wash the wound and remove all traces of the venom.
☆ Take the child to a doctor immediately keeping the limb as still as possible. It is helpful if you can remember what the snake looked like.

Stings

Stings are very painful in the short term so plenty of cuddles are needed. Antihistamine creams are available from the chemist which are handy to have available during the summer. If your child has a severe reaction to a sting take him immediately to the doctor particularly if he is stung in the mouth. Shock can also occur and needs emergency treatment. The child will appear pale, sweaty and faint – do not delay in seeking help.

BLACK EYE

Any hard blow around the eyebrow, nose or cheek may result in swelling and later a black eye. As the eye is well set back in the socket, it is unlikely to be damaged. If you fear that there has been some injury, take the child to the doctor who may be able to examine the eye, although in many cases this is impossible because of the swelling. A cold compress such as a flannel or a tea towel wrapped round a bag of frozen peas, will help soothe the pain. Black eyes usually become less swollen after a few days, becoming yellowy as they fade.

BLEEDING

Children are usually very frightened by bleeding so be calm and reassuring. Tell them that the blood is cleaning the cut.

Heavy bleeding: Blood which is dripping rather than oozing needs to be controlled quickly. Pressure applied to seal the cut edges will form a clot on the cut and stop the flow of blood. If the blood spurts from the wound:

☆ Press hard on the wound and raise the limb above the heart level if possible (unless the limb appears broken).

☆ If the blood still spurts out try to find a bone to press the cut against. Once you have found a place that will reduce or stop the flow, DO NOT MOVE YOUR FINGERS. If the wound is on the trunk, lie the child down and use your closed fist to press the wound against a bone.

☆ Get help by shouting or carrying the child to help if this is possible. If you have to leave the child try to replace the pressure with something hard and heavy. DO NOT REMOVE ANY OBJECT STICKING OUT OF THE WOUND. DO NOT GIVE THE CHILD ANYTHING TO EAT OR DRINK IN CASE AN OPERATION IS REQUIRED. The child may suffer from shock.

Light bleeding: Usually light bleeding will stop as a clot forms. If it does not, press it firmly with a pad of clean gauze or cotton for up to ten minutes. Replace pad with a sticking plaster or a sterile dressing.

PRECAUTION:

Is your child up to date with tetanus immunisation? See page 40. He may be at risk.

BURNS AND SCALDS

Burns do not only affect the skin that you can see. The heat can cause plasma in the blood vessels to escape causing a blister. A severe burn that removes the skin will therefore remove a large amount of plasma from the child's circulation and can cause shock. The severity of a burn should therefore be judged by the area it covers rather than its depth. Sometimes the plasma will need to be replaced by fluids in the hospital.

✫ If the burn becomes infected, more painful or oozes fluid or pus, see your doctor.

Burns can be caused by fire, chemicals, electricity and hot objects. Scalds are caused by hot liquids and steam. Burns and scalds hurt more than any other wound.

Action
1. Take child away from the object that has burnt or scalded him.
2. Cool the area for ten minutes under cold NOT ICED running water. DO NOT USE A SHOWER.
3. Take off clothing or jewellery as swelling may later make this difficult.
4. If the burn is less than 2 cm (¾ in) square it can be treated at home. If it is larger it should be seen by a doctor especially if it is on the face, hands, soles of feet, genital area or a joint.

5. Wrap the burn in a clean handkerchief or sheet to keep infection away from the raw skin. Call an ambulance or get him to hospital quickly.
6. If the burn can be treated at home:
   ☆ Dry the area gently — do not use cotton wool.
   ☆ Leave any blisters alone as the area is then protected from infection and plasma is unable to leak further.
   ☆ Put on a sterile adhesive dressing to protect it or put on sterile gauze and a bandage to keep it in place.
   ☆ DO NOT APPLY ANY OINTMENT.
   ☆ The child may suffer from shock.

Scald in the Mouth

Try to get the child to suck some ice or eat an ice cream. Water sipped through a straw is also a good way of cooling the specific part of the mouth that has been damaged.

Avoid acid foods and serve food lukewarm for the following few days until the scald has healed.

Electrical Burns

PRECAUTION

Remember to TURN OFF THE SOURCE OF ELEC-TRICITY BEFORE TOUCHING THE CHILD.

Like scalds there may be little to see on the skin's surface after an electrical burn. There will be a blackened spot where the current entered but not blistered.

Take the child to the doctor immediately as the flesh

under the skin may well be damaged as the current fanned out.

Clothes on Fire
1. Provided the fire does not involve electricity or oil soak the clothes with water.
2. If oil is involved or no water is available cover the child in a rug, curtain or similar object to smother the flames. DO NOT USE SYNTHETIC FABRICS AND DO NOT ROLL THE CHILD.
3. If nothing is available, cover the flames with your own body to prevent air fanning the blaze.

EYE INJURIES

Any injury or accident involving the eye ball should be seen by a doctor. Do not delay, even the tiniest scratch can become infected or cause loss of vision however temporary. Cover the eye as long as it does not make the child more frightened.

Corrosive or stinging liquid in the eye
Shampoo or soap can cause a great deal of irritation if it gets in the eye. It will not cause any lasting damage though it does hurt at the time.

For any other liquid
Wash the eye continuously under a gently running tap, or use a jug making sure that the water flows away from the good eye. Go on for about ten minutes ignoring protests as, if it is an acid or alkali, *his sight may be at stake*.

Telephone the doctor to see whether he needs to be seen at the casualty department for the eye to be irrigated. Take the container of irritant with you.

Foreign body in the eye
Usually minor irritants such as dust, sand or an insect

will be washed out by the tears, crying will therefore help. Try not to let the child rub his eye, it is better that he blinks and blows his nose. Standing behind him in a good light, separate the eye lids and see if you can see the object. If you can you may be able to flush it out with a little cold water dripped over the eye from a syringe or small cup.

PRECAUTIONS

☆ Do not use any sharp object such as tweezers to remove an irritant from the eye.

☆ Do not try to remove anything from the coloured part of the eye.

☆ Do not try to remove anything that seems stuck to the surface of the eye.

☆ Be careful about using a tissue or hanky to remove a foreign body from the eye as it can damage the eye.

☆ If you have nothing else available you can use your tongue to sweep over the eyeball.

CHOKING

Children can choke on very small things, so for this reason it is not advisable to leave them alone to eat especially when young. Usually coughing will bring up the object. If the child can cough it means that some air must be getting through. If he is turning blue then it is an emergency.

☆ Check to see if you can see the object. See if you can hook it out with your finger. By making him sick the object may also be dislodged.

✰ Put him across your knees with his head lower than his legs and pat him firmly between the shoulder blades.

✰ If the object has still not moved call an ambulance or rush him to hospital in the head down position banging his back all the time if you can.

CONVULSIONS

Convulsions are caused by a sudden rise in the temperature of a young baby or child. The child will become rigid and then the muscles will clench and unclench with jerks and twitches. Convulsions are very frightening especially because they often start when you pick the child up or touch him because you are worried at his strange expressions and twitching.

✰ Do not leave him if you can avoid it. Get someone else to phone for help.

✰ Take care to ensure he does not inhale any vomit.

✰ Try to keep him on his side or on his front with his head turned to one side.

✰ Do not restrain him.

✰ Do not touch his mouth except to remove vomit.

Usually convulsions only last a few minutes. Children usually fall into a deep sleep afterwards. Treat him for the high temperature by tepid sponging to help him cool down. See page 18.

DISLOCATIONS

Dislocations occur when the ball part of the joint comes out of its socket. Usually dislocations are accompanied by fractures, however shoulders and jaws can dislocate without a fracture. The diagnosis of dislocation needs to be carried out by a doctor, with an X-ray to confirm the diagnosis. It is best if treatment is begun within 3 hours of the accident before swelling starts.

☆ The child will be in great pain. Sometimes jaw dislocations go back of their own accord as the child cries out. Treatment will then not be necessary.

☆ Put the dislocated shoulder in a sling with the arm across the chest.

☆ DO NOT GIVE THE CHILD ANYTHING TO EAT OR DRINK AS HE MAY NEED AN ANAESTHETIC.

☆ Take him straight to hospital.

DROWNING

If your child falls into a swimming pool and you can swim — leap in to rescue him. If the water is dangerous, shout for help first.

☆ See if there is a lifebelt, rope, boat or bridge near that might help you.

☆ In moving water jump ahead of the child, having looked at the flow of the water, so that he will come towards you.

☆ Always stay with a boat that has capsized — you will be more easily seen and the boat will provide some support.

☆ Lilos can be very dangerous in the sea. Tell the child to stay on the lilo or boat whilst you get help. Always alert someone before you attempt to rescue the child so that you can also be watched.

☆ If your child appears to have inhaled a lot of water and is not breathing start the kiss of life. If you are unable to do this put him over your shoulder and go for help.

☆ If he is coughing and vomiting, then he is breathing. Put him in the recovery position on his side with one knee drawn up and one arm behind his back — then get help.

FOREIGN BODY IN THE EAR OR NOSE

Leave the object alone as you may push it in even
further and cause damage. Take the child to a doctor to
have it removed.

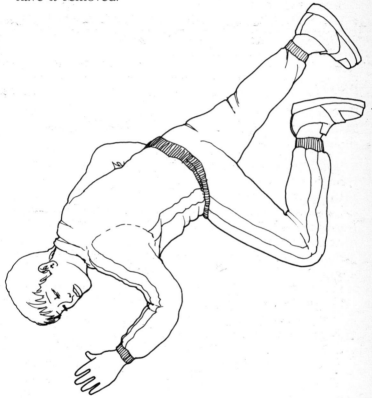

FRACTURES

Greenstick fractures occur in young children. The child
will complain of pain and the limb may be swollen. The
child will be reluctant to use it. Take the child to the
doctor for examination and X-ray, having put the limb in

a comfortable postion. *Do not give him anything to eat or drink* as he may need an anaesthetic. If the child seems to be in shock it is more likely that he has sustained a severe fracture particularly if he is unable to move the limb.

* Don't move him unless you are certain that he has not damaged his pelvis (hip bone) or spine. Call for an ambulance. Movement will possibly damage the injury further so try to keep him and the damaged limb still.
* Use a stretcher to carry him, or make one with a coat or a removable car seat.
* If the skin is broken, cover the area with a clean dressing. Do not attempt to clean the wound as you may introduce infection.

HEAD INJURY

It is important to observe your child carefully if he has hit his head or fallen. Put an ice pack or bag of frozen vegetables on the bump to ease the swelling.

* If he seems dazed, lay him down and watch him. If he sleeps check that his colour and breathing are normal. If he stays pale or becomes paler and starts to breathe harshly, wake him up. If he is easy to wake then don't worry, but if he cannot be roused, call for a doctor.

* The vital signs to watch for are:
Vomiting
Eye peculiarities
Mumbled or irrational speech
Bleeding
Headache which continues
Clumsiness
Failure to recognize you

In this situation call for a doctor immediately.

NOSEBLEEDS

Children are usually terrified by the sight of blood so try to wash as much of it away as possible.

☆ If the bleeding is heavy, pinch the nostrils firmly for 2 minutes so that the blood has a chance to clot.
☆ Once the bleeding has stopped, don't let the child blow or pick his nose for at least an hour. The nose will feel uncomfortable and crusty.

POISONING

A child that has eaten or drunk poison must be treated very quickly.

☆ Clear his mouth of any tablets.
☆ Check for the container so that you can say how much has been swallowed, take it with you to the casualty department.
☆ Some poisons should not be vomited up as they will cause further burning.
☆ Rush the child to hospital as quickly as possible.

SPLINTERS

Many splinters can be removed using tweezers. If you cannot see which way it went in, it may be possible to squeeze it out or help it out with a sterilised needle.

☆ If the splinter is not painful leave it alone as it will make its own way out in time.
☆ Glass or metal splinters should be removed by a doctor.

SWALLOWED OBJECTS

Most objects that a child may swallow will probably do no harm. If the object is sharp or contains cotton wool he will need medical attention.

☆ Check the mouth and hands for the object before you rush him to hospital.

UNCONSCIOUSNESS

Any child who is unconscious needs medical help immediately.

☆ Check that he cannot choke and help his circulation by getting him into the recovery position.

☆ Lie him on his tummy with his head turned to one side.

☆ Draw the leg on that side well up, with his arm bent at the elbow so the hand is opposite the face.

☆ Vomit or blood is now able to drain out without obstructing the breathing. Do not try to give him anything to drink.

☆ If he regains consciousness keep him lying down until the doctor arrives. (See Recovery Position, page 33).

Despite all the care and attention that you pay to your child, accidents do still happen so it is worth finding out about first aid so that you are prepared. It may not be your own child who needs your help, but a child in your care or a neighbour perhaps. The St John's Ambulance, British Red Cross Society and Royal Life Saving Society all run courses which the public are encouraged to attend. Ask at your local library for details. Here you will learn basic first aid, how to give the kiss of life if breathing has stopped and how to give heart massage.

Local knowledge is also important. Do you know

where your nearest casualty department is? If you haven't a telephone where is the nearest? All this information should be written down and preferably kept near the telephone or on the medicine cupboard door.

Information to have to hand

Name of doctor:

Telephone:

Address:

Name of nearest hospital with casualty department:

Hours of opening:

Relative or neighbour to be contacted in an emergency:

Chapter 5

IMMUNISATION AND THE PREVENTION OF INFECTIOUS DISEASES

All babies in Britain are offered protection against seven potentially devastating illnesses: diphtheria, tetanus, whooping cough, polio, measles, mumps and rubella or German measles. Although the timing of immunisations against these diseases may vary from area to area, in general they follow this pattern:

2 months: diphtheria, tetanus, whooping cough and polio
3 months: diphtheria, tetanus, whooping cough and polio
4 months: diphtheria, tetanus, whooping cough and polio
12–15 months: measles, mumps and rubella
5 years or school entry: diphtheria, tetanus and polio

It is vital that your baby is given these immunisations because it means that he probably will not then get these diseases or if he does, it will only be in a very mild form and not life threatening. Every year babies and young children still die from these diseases because their parents have decided against having them protected by the injections.

A great deal has been written in the newspapers and

in magazines about the so-called dangers of immunisation, but the risk of death or serious illness from the disease is far greater than the risks arising from immunisation. Nevertheless your health visitor and doctor will understand your concerns and will be happy to talk to you. Some parents believe that because no one these days seems to catch diphtheria or polio there is no need for their baby to be immunised. These illnesses have only become rare because of the large number of parents who do have their babies protected. If these numbers fall, then we will see a rise in these often fatal infections. They are certainly not yet extinct like smallpox, which is not routinely given now as an immunisation as the risk of the vaccine is greater than the risk of contracting the disease. It is expected that smallpox will be completely eradicated from the world in the near future.

Most parents do not remember or were not born when these diseases were common and are unaware of how ill many children became. There are still people living today who depend on an iron lung to keep them alive because they had polio as a child. There is also an increased risk of contracting these diseases when travelling abroad.

Immunity to disease can be acquired by getting the disease itself or by immunisation. Once a child has actually suffered from an infection he will have developed his own antibodies to it and will be unlikely to get it again. With the diseases that can be prevented by immunisation, it is safer to build up the child's antibodies before he comes in contact with the infection. Immunisations can either be active where the child is given a weak form of the organisms that cause the disease so that he makes his own antibodies, or passive where antibodies are actually given to the child by immunisation.

FIRST IMMUNISATIONS

DIPHTHERIA

Diphtheria was once a dangerous disease which needed urgent treatment by a doctor so that complications did not occur.

Progress of the disease: The disease started in the throat making a grey-coloured membrane over the tonsils. The child would start to feel very ill but would not have a temperature. Occasionally the disease would start in the nose causing a bloody discharge. As the disease progressed the larynx or voice box was affected and breathing became more and more difficult until emergency treatment was needed. The disease produces harmful poisons which attack the heart and nervous system. The **treatment** of diphtheria is by giving diphtheria anti-toxin and antibiotics but needs to be started early if it is to be successul. Once the child has recovered he will need the full course of immunisation as he will still not have long-lasting immunity. Immunisation against diphtheria is always given together with tetanus and usually whooping cough. Booster doses are given at five years of age and then every ten years.

TETANUS

Tetanus or lockjaw is caused by a bacterium that produces spasms of muscles in the neck and jaw. Each year several hundred people in Britain get tetanus and some of them die.

Tetanus is caused by an infection of a cut or wound which is fairly deep. Horse manure is one of the most common sources of tetanus infection which means that gardeners and stable workers are particularly at risk. A prick from a rose thorn that is infected can be enough to cause the disease and be fatal. Tetanus can also be found in dust around the house.

Progress of the disease: Once the tetanus bacteria is in the body, toxins or poisons are produced which travel in the blood to the brain. It may take up to six months for any symptoms to start so the diagnosis of tetanus is often difficult. The disease starts with a sore throat, followed by pain in the muscles particularly around the neck. The next stage is the start of spasms of the mouth and jaw and later if the disease is not treated, the rest of the body will become affected and the person may die in severe cases.

Treatment: If you suspect that your child may have cut or pricked himself on something that may be infected you should discuss your child's immunity with your doctor. If he has had the course of immunisation as a baby he may be given a booster dose of vaccine. If he has not had the immunisations he will need a dose of anti-tetanus globulin which will protect him against the toxins. This needs to be given as quickly as possible.

The best protection from tetanus is prevention by immunising your baby. Booster doses are given at five years of age and then every five to ten years.

WHOOPING COUGH

Whooping cough is still a serious problem in Britain which can cause death in up to 40% of infected babies. It is highly infectious and easily spread especially amongst pre-school age children. Adults can also get the infection as immunity from this disease does not last for life.

The bacilli which cause whooping cough, or pertussis as it is also known, are spread by coughing or breathing out infected droplets which are then inhaled by another person. The incubation time for the disease is between one and two weeks with the child being infectious before the disease is even noticed. Whooping cough normally lasts for six to eight weeks and needs a great deal of nursing care with resulting lack of sleep for the parent.

Progress of the disease: The disease starts with what appears to be a cold accompanied by a slightly raised temperature and a cough. It moves on to the characteristic 'whoop' which is a bout of coughing followed by the intake of air through the partially closed windpipe. These whoops may occur infrequently or more than a hundred times a day. Vomiting may accompany the coughing especially in young babies. Babies may stop breathing and may have a convulsion.

The last stage of the illness is the convalescent period which may last up to three weeks. During this time the child must be kept isolated until the coughing stops to prevent further infection of others.

Treatment: Sometimes medicine containing atropine is given to help control the muscle spasm during the coughing bout. Cough mixtures do not seem to help at all. Breast-fed babies can be fed if the feed is started at the beginning of the bout of coughing as this seems to help and reduces the risk of vomiting later. If the coughing is really disturbing the child (and family) at night some sedatives may be given. Occasionally antibiotics are given if pneumonia is suspected. Pneumonia and other lung diseases are the main cause of death in these babies. Otitis media (ear infection) and convulsions can also occur.

Babies over five months seem to recover completely. Usually, it is the smaller ones who are most vulnerable. This is because of their immature lungs and the need for frequent feeds to maintain adequate growth and development and avoid the subsequent danger of dehydration. Very small babies are often taken in to hospital as it is thought that complications will be picked up and treated earlier.

The Department of Health recommend immunisation against whooping cough for all babies unless otherwise advised by your doctor.

POLIO

Polio is an infection of the spinal cord that is caused by three viruses. It is found in the stools and saliva of infected people and is transmitted by direct contact or contamination of toys, food or swimming pools.

Progress of the disease: From the moment of infection the virus takes up to two weeks to develop. The majority of children who develop polio will have no symptoms and will just become immune, of the remainder, 5% will have minor symptoms of sore throat, fever and nausea for a few days and 1–2% will develop full-blown polio. This has the previous symptoms as well as sore stiff muscles, a stiff neck and spine and general malaise. Of the children contracting polio, about 1% will become paralysed and may die.

Treatment: The diagnosis of polio will need to be confirmed by a doctor using blood samples. Pain killers will be given or hot packs to relieve the pain and stiffness. If paralysis occurs, the danger is that the respiratory muscles may be involved, resulting in difficulty in breathing. The treatment for this is for the child to be put in a respirator. Physiotherapy will be needed to prevent the paralysed limbs becoming deformed.

Obviously the prevention of the disease is of prime

importance and this is done by giving vaccine by mouth in the first four months of life with a booster dose at five years. If your baby vomits within an hour of the vaccine he may not be fully protected and may need a repeat dose. For this reason it is sensible to have your baby immunised about two hours after a feed.

Breast-fed babies will be protected from polio during the early weeks but should still receive the vaccine. Polio is still common particularly in hot countries. It is therefore worthwhile making sure that your child is fully immunised if you are considering travelling beyond Northern Europe or Canada and the USA.

PRACTICAL POINTERS TO REMEMBER

☆ Talk about immunisation with your partner, health visitor or GP.

☆ Dress your baby sensibly when going for the immunisation to allow clothes to be removed easily.

☆ Feed your baby about two hours before the immunisation if possible.

☆ The immunisation is usually given in the arm or leg. There may be a little redness for a few days and occasionally a lump may appear. This is nothing to worry about.

☆ Keep infant paracetamol to hand if your baby becomes feverish and is over four months old.

☆ Report any side effects to your doctor or health visitor.

MEASLES, MUMPS AND RUBELLA

Between 12 and 15 months your child will have the opportunity to have the MMR vaccine. This offers protection against measles, mumps and rubella (German measles). Twenty years ago children commonly caught these infections and many suffered serious side effects such as encephalitis, pneumonia and bronchitis. It is now possible to prevent them by one injection in childhood. Hopefully during the next ten years, these diseases, like diphtheria, will become rare. All of this group of infectious diseases is harmful to adults who have not been immunised.

MEASLES

Measles is a very infectious disease that occurs in epidemics. It is passed from child to child by an airborne or droplet virus. It has an incubation period of 10–12 days following exposure to the virus, and can be passed on to others well before any rash appears.

Progress of the illness: The first symptoms of measles are those of a cold with a runny nose, sore eyes and a fever, often there is a cough too. During these early stages there are small white spots inside the cheeks near the back molars. As the cough and temperature get worse, a heavy red rash appears first behind the ears and then on the neck and face. The rash spreads all over the trunk of the child and occasionally on to the arms and legs. The rash will last for three or four days and, as it fades, so the temperature will disappear and the child will recover. The side effects of measles are severe earache, possible broncho-pneumonia when the cough becomes severe together with a high fever and, most serious of all, encephalitis or inflammation of the brain. With encephalitis the child becomes drowsy, nauseous and has a severe headache. All of these side effects need treatment immediately from your doctor.

Treatment: A normal attack of measles needs no special treatment from the doctor. Encourage plenty of cool drinks, light meals and plenty of rest. Keep him away from bright light.

In the case of side effects or complications, antibiotics may be prescribed. If the child's eyes are sore they can be bathed in warm slightly salt water. The fever can be controlled by paracetamol syrup and the cough eased by a suppressant cough mixture if necessary.

PRECAUTIONS

* ☆ Make sure your child is completely recovered before he returns to playgroup, nursery or school. He will be likely to pick up any other infections that are around.
* ☆ Check that all signs of the rash have gone before he mixes with others as he will still be infectious whilst he has the rash.
* ☆ Breast-fed babies are unlikely to catch measles in the first six months of life if the mother has had the infection.
* ☆ Immunisation can be given at any age. If your child has been in contact with measles and has not been immunised, your doctor may give him an injection of gammaglobulin to help prevent the measles.
* ☆ Immunisation protection against measles is not lifelong — children over eleven years may sometimes have a mild attack of measles which should clear rapidly.

MUMPS

Mumps is caused by a virus infection of the salivary glands. It is usually caught by coming into contact with the saliva of someone already infected. It is unusual for children under the age of five to contract the disease. The disease takes two to three weeks to incubate.

Progress of the disease: After the incubation period the child will start to feel unwell and will have a fever and muscular pains in the neck. He may also complain of a headache and be reluctant to eat. Young children with the disease will complain of a swelling in front of one ear. The other side may swell a few days later, but this is not always the case. Glands under the jaw will become swollen and the child's mouth will be dry. The child will find it difficult to eat, drink and speak and sour drinks or condiments such as lemon juice, salad dressing or vinegar will make it more painful. The swellings last from seven to fourteen days, with the child being generally irritable and off-colour and in pain. Complications of mumps include encephalitis and deafness. The disease can also affect the ovaries and testes or cause infection of the pancreas.

PRECAUTIONS

☆ If a mother has had mumps a baby will be immune from the disease for 4–6 months.

☆ Mumps can be immunised against at any time.

☆ Mumps in teenage boys and men rarely causes sterility but can cause considerable pain. Infertility is rarely caused by mumps in women.

☆ If your child is sick, complains of a headache and appears drowsy he may have an inflammation of the brain called encephalitis. If you are worried and think he may have this, call your doctor at once.

Treatment: There is no specific drug treatment for mumps so each individual symptom needs to be looked at. Food should be soft and mashed and drinks given regularly using a straw. After meals give the child a mouthwash or brush his teeth as gum infections can occur. Keep the child isolated from others particularly adults who have not had the disease. Paracetamol can be given to reduce the temperature. Where there are complications the doctor may prescribe treatment. Keep the child at home until the swelling has gone down.

RUBELLA OR GERMAN MEASLES

German measles or rubella is usually a very mild infectious disease. It can be transmitted by droplets of sputum on coughing, and by direct contact with items such as cups or spoons that the infected person has used or by items in contact with nose, throat, urine or stools. The incubation period is 14–21 days. Once a child has had German measles he will be immune for life.

Progress of the disease: The first sign of German measles will usually be a mild catarrh. The lymph nodes at the back of the neck and behind the ears will become swollen and tender. A few days later a rash starts from behind the ears and on the forehead and spreads over the body. The rash usually lasts for two or three days and the child may have a slight fever. The throat is usually rather dry and red and consequently the child may not be very interested in eating. There may be some itching from the rash and earache is also quite common. Joint pain is sometimes experienced by older girls, but this will disappear in about two weeks. The child should be kept isolated for at least four days after the rash has disappeared.

Treatment: Paracetamol can be given to reduce the fever and help joint pain, otherwise there is usually no need to give any other medicine. It is a good idea to have the diagnosis of German measles confirmed by a doctor if your child has not been immunised.

PRECAUTIONS

☆ Rubella immunisation is offered to all 10–11-year-old girls at present until the Department of Health feel that enough babies are being immunised to prevent the epidemics of rubella that can be so devastating to the baby of a newly pregnant woman.

☆ Rubella immunisation can be given at any time following a blood test to check whether the person is immune. Women who wish to become pregnant should be immunised at least two months before conceiving a baby.

☆ If a woman who has not been immunised against rubella contracts the disease in the first three months of pregnancy she may have a miscarriage. In some cases the pregnancy will continue and the baby runs the risk of being born with cataracts, deafness or a heart defect. A pregnant woman in this situation should discuss her options with her doctor immediately.

☆ Babies are protected against rubella if the mother herself is immune. Antibodies will pass across the placenta and protect the baby.

HIV INFECTION

It is extremely rare for children to be in circumstances where they could pick up the infection; however, a baby born to a mother who is HIV positive will itself be HIV positive, although possibly not infected. A further test is done at 18 months.

The need for help and advice is every parent's right, together with the need for privacy and confidentiality. The relationship between parent and child can suffer once the diagnosis has been made, so contact with support groups is vital. Ask your GP or health visitor for the names of local groups who will be able to help.

The National Children's Bureau (8 Wakley Street, London, EC1V 7QE, tel: 071–278 9441) can give information about organisations concerned with HIV infection. The local Health Education Department should also have local information.

Chapter 6

AT-A-GLANCE GUIDE TO THE COMMON INFECTIOUS DISEASES

DISEASE	SYMPTOMS	INCUBATION	TREATMENT	COMPLICATIONS	ISOLATION	PREVENTION
Chicken-pox	Headache, fever, swollen lymph nodes, blotchy rash which 2 days later appears as small pimples over trunk. After few hours they blister, then dry and fall off after about 10 days unless them become infected.	17–21 days	Calamine lotion will help soothe the itchy spots. Keep finger nails short so that the spots are not scratched so easily. Occasionally sedatives may be prescribed if child cannot sleep.	Occasionally children have a really bad rash which may cover the inside of the mouth, vagina, anus, ears and scalp. An ointment can be prescribed to help spots particularly in the genital area. Encephalitis is a rare complication of chicken pox.	Keep away from other children until all the scabs have dried.	No immunisation yet available. Chicken-pox is dangerous to young babies and those on steroids or other immuno-suppressant drugs. Chicken-pox virus can cause shingles in an adult and vice versa.
Fifth Disease (Slapped Cheek Syndrome)	A reddened cheek and blotchy rash on arms, trunk and lower parts of the legs. The rash is itchy and gets worse if the child gets	7–28 days	Any fever can be treated with paracetamol and the itching if intense can be helped with antihistamines. Keep child cool.	No complications.	No isolation necessary.	None.

overheated. The rash may last up to 5 weeks but usually goes after about 11 days, fading away to a lace-like rash.

German measles (Rubella)	Cold, sore throat, slight temperature, tiredness, lack of appetite, conjunctivitis, swollen lymph glands. 1 day later rash of pink slightly raised spots which appear blotchy, behind ears, on forehead and spreading to rest of body. Itchy rash which disappears quickly.	2–3 weeks	May need something to suck to soothe the sore throat. Keep out of sunlight and away from heat which may make rash itch more.	None to the child itself but may damage an unborn baby by causing deafness, heart disorder or cataracts.	Keep away from all pregnant women for 1 week before the rash appears to 8 days after it has gone.	Immunisation at 12–15 months. Tell any women your child has been in contact with whilst infectious.

DISEASE	SYMPTOMS	INCUBATION	TREATMENT	COMPLICATIONS	ISOLATION	PREVENTION
Measles	Slight temperature, white spots in mouth, dry cough and cold, sore eyes, tummy ache, swollen lymph glands. Rash spreads from behind ears and over upper half of body. Diarrhoea and vomiting.	10–12 days	Paracetamol, cough medicine. Plenty of drinks.	Antibiotics may be needed for ear infection. Bronchitis, pneumonia and occasionally encephalitis.	Keep away from non-immune children from 7 days after exposure until 10 days after rash begins.	Immunisation at 12–15 months.
Mumps	General feeling of being unwell. Fever, headache, muscle swelling and pain especially in front of ears. Dry mouth and pain on eating.	2–3 weeks	Give plenty of drinks and keep mouth clean by tooth brushing and mouthwashes. Mash food and avoid lemon and acid foods.	Meningitis, encephalitis and inflammation of the pancreas.	Infectious from 6 days before swelling to 3 days after swelling has gone.	Immunisation at 12–15 months.

	Symptoms	Incubation	Treatment	Complications	Infectious period	Notes
Roseola Infantum	A rapid high fever with accompanying sore throat, cold and headache. A rash appears as flat spots or pimples on trunk, neck, arms, face and legs.	7–17 days	Keep child cool and treat fever with paracetamol which will also help the sore throat.	Sometimes children have convulsions. The disease should not be confused with German measles.	None necessary.	This infection only usually seen in children of 6–24 months. It usually occurs in spring and autumn.
Scarlet Fever	Sudden fever, headache, vomiting, loss of appetite, tummy ache and swollen lymph glands followed by a rash of small red spots which feel rough. These spread over trunk but are seldom seen round the mouth. Gradually fading to flaky skin. Tongue very coated and sore throat.	1–7 days	Antibiotics, light diet and plenty of drinks.	Otitis media or middle ear infection. Kidney infection though this is fairly rare now because of early use of antibiotics. Rheumatic fever also is rarely seen now as a complication.	Infectious for up to 2 days after start of antibiotics.	The child's urine should be checked after the illness for infection.

DISEASE	SYMPTOMS	INCUBATION	TREATMENT	COMPLICATIONS	ISOLATION	PREVENTION
Whooping Cough	Starts with a cold which leads to a cough often with the classic 'whoop'. Vomiting and weight loss especially in babies. Blueness of skin and sometimes convulsions.	8–14 days	Breast-feeding helps. Antibiotics may be prescribed which will shorten the length of isolation period. Sedatives can be given in cases of sleeplessness.	Convulsions, pneumonia, ear infection.	7 days if child is given antibiotics — otherwise 21 days.	Immunisation at 2, 3 and 4 months.

Chapter 7

THE SKIN AND ASSOCIATED PROBLEMS

The skin protects our bodies from infection, injury and extremes of weather. It is regularly renewed every 28

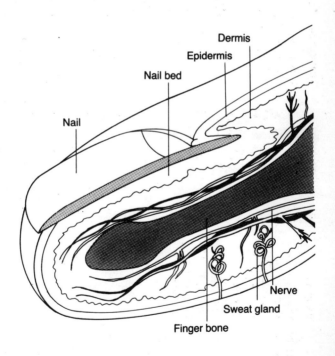

days as the dead flattened cells of the outer layer (epidermis) flake off through daily wear and tear. Within the epidermis is the pigment melanin which gives us our skin colour.

Underneath the epidermis is the dermis which contains elastic fibres, protein and collagen and a very good nerve supply which responds if necessary to touch, temperature and pain. Sweat is manufactured in the dermis and acts as an antiseptic and coolant for the body. It is also a means of removing waste products. Deep in the dermis are also found the hair follicles.

The skin also acts as an indicator of general bodily health and well-being. Signs of illness may include swelling or puffiness, redness or blueness, feeling hot or cold, dryness or dampness, or appearing pale, pigmented or covered in a rash.

AN A–Z OF COMMON SKIN CONDITIONS

CONDITION

TREATMENT

ABSCESS

This usually is identified by a sore reddened area which contains a collection of pus. If it has been present for a while the child may have a slight fever.

Needs to be seen by a doctor to remove the pus and give antibiotics if necessary. Sometimes abscesses are a sign of general ill health.

ALLERGY

An allergy to a food or substance can sometimes be seen on the skin as a rash.

Itchiness can sometimes be relieved by calamine lotion or antihistamine on prescription.

CONDITION

TREATMENT

Try to work out what caused the allergy and avoid it where possible. If concerned see your health visitor or GP.

ANAEMIA

Iron deficiency in the blood seen as paleness of skin especially of lower eyelid.

Needs to be treated by a doctor to find out the cause. Iron tablets may be given or you may be advised on your child's diet. A blood test will be taken.

ANAL FISSURE

A crack in the skin around the anus which is painful and may bleed.

Keep the anal area soft and lubricated with petroleum jelly. Increase fibre in the diet (cereals, fruit and vegetables) and encourage extra drinks as constipation makes it more painful.

ATHLETE'S FOOT

Itching, scaling and cracking between the toes caused by a fungus that grows well in moist conditions.

Fungicidal ointment should be applied daily to clean dry feet. Discourage use of trainers and other rubber soled shoes. Highly infectious.

BALANITIS

Inflammation of the end of the penis. The foreskin is infected by a secretion or an irritant such as sand.

The foreskin should be gently retracted and the penis well washed. A little antiseptic cream will aid healing. Repeat this

CONDITION

TREATMENT

twice daily. If there is no improvement the doctor may prescribe antibiotics.

BALDNESS

Can be caused by ringworm, rubbing or pulling out resulting in bald spots or alopecia areata which is more long-lasting and is difficult to treat.

Baldness caused by ringworm can easily be treated with ointment from your doctor. Children who pull out their hair may be worried about something. Have a chat to your health visitor or doctor if you are concerned.

BIRTHMARKS

Most birthmarks are harmless and many fade as the child gets older. The port wine stain will remain but strawberry naevi which appears a few days after birth will disappear by about two years.

Ask the paediatrician or doctor about the birthmark if you are worried. Make-up is available if the birthmark makes the child self-conscious.

BITES AND STINGS – see page 71

BLISTERS

Blisters on the skin can be caused by severe sunburn, cold sores, allergic reactions especially to plants and burns. They are also caused by friction as with ill-fitting shoes.

Try to leave the blisters alone as this will decrease the risk of infecting the new skin underneath. Keep them uncovered if possible especially at night.

BLUENESS

Usually caused by not enough oxygen circulating in the blood.

Many small babies have blue fingers and toes even though

CONDITION

TREATMENT

they appear warm. This is caused by the immaturity of their circulatory system and will improve. There are some heart defects which are usually identified at birth which can cause blueness. If you notice that your baby suddenly looks blue you should ask your doctor to examine him.

BOILS

Boils are small infections which occur beneath the skin often in hair follicles. They contain infected pus.

Boils come to a head easily if soaked in Epsom Salts. Once the boil bursts be careful to wash away all pus from the area and keep the surrounding skin clean. Never squeeze a boil as the infection may spread. Your doctor may drain the boil if it does not come to a head of its own accord. Antibiotics may be given.

BRUISES

Bruises are caused by damage to small blood vessels in the skin. The colour comes from the pooling of blood near the surface. They can be caused by fighting amongst children and physical abuse of children. They are also a sign of possible haemophilia and sometimes leukaemia if there is no obvious cause.

Leaving the affected part under the cold tap or using an icepack for 10–15 minutes will help lessen bruising after an accident. The bruise may take a day or two to come out and often up to a week to fade. If you are concerned that your child gets more bruises than you might expect, speak to your doctor.

CONDITION   TREATMENT

CHAPPED SKIN/CRACKED LIPS

Can be caused by ill health and accompanying high temperature. Extremes of temperatures and allergy to foods can also result in chapped skin and lips.

Chapped skin can be very painful and should be protected by a cream, lipsalve or petroleum jelly. Advise your child not to lick the lips as it makes it worse.

CHICKEN-POX — see page 52

CHILBLAINS

Caused by not wearing enough warm clothing in cold weather. The chilblains appear as swollen, red, itchy and painful areas on the hands or feet.

Keep the skin warm and apply arnica tincture if it is painful. Encourage the child to exercise the hands and feet to improve the circulation and make sure that he is well wrapped up in cold weather.

COLD SORES

Caused by the virus herpes simplex and are usually seen round the mouth. The virus will reappear as a result of stress, fever and extremes of temperature.

Cold sores are like blisters which are extremely itchy. If scratched they may become infected. Usually they respond to creams available from the chemist, but if they become a problem see your doctor.

CRADLE CAP — see seborrhoeic dermatitis page 70

DANDRUFF

White flakes of skin which is normal in small amounts but if in larger amounts it may be caused by over production of oil in the skin.

Use a mild shampoo for children's hair. Medicated shampoos can be used if the problem persists. Ask your health visitor to recommend one.

CONDITION

ECZEMA

The most common type of eczema, 'atopic' eczema, runs in families who are prone to hayfever, asthma or other allergies. There is often no cause found for it, and the majority of children cease to have it by the time they are three. Eczema can also be caused by irritant substances such as plants, citrus fruits, detergents and bubblebaths, soap and some drugs. It usually begins on the face with red scaly patches which are very itchy. It is often found behind the ears and will spread to all the moist creases of the body. If the child scratches the skin, it will itch even more. The blisters will form crusts from the oozing fluid and they may become infected. Contact eczema only affects the area that has been in contact with the irritant.

TREATMENT

Atopic eczema has no cure but there are many things which may help.

☆ Bath baby less frequently and use a mineral oil instead of soap.

☆ Try to choose cotton clothes — sweating and itchiness makes eczema worse.

☆ Wash clothes and nappies well in mild washing powder and rinse without fabric conditioner.

☆ Try to find out what is causing contact eczema and avoid it, but beware of rotation diets unless supervised by a dietician. Patch testing is also of doubtful value.

☆ Occasionally eczema is caused by an allergy to cow's milk. Ask your GP about it if you suspect this may be the cause.

☆ Stress such as separation from home or entry to a day nursery may make the eczema worse.

☆ Keep fingernails clean and short. Creams may be prescribed if the conditions becomes severe.

☆ Talk to parents of other children with eczema. Your health visitor may be able to put you in touch. The National Eczema

CONDITION

TREATMENT

Society (see page 124) also has many useful leaflets and is a good source of advice. Eczema can be a very distressing and exhausting condition for both parents and children.

HEAT RASH

Usually caused by overwrapping a baby or exposure to sunlight which causes a similar itchy rash often called prickly heat. The rash is made up of raised pink spots over chest, neck and shoulders which are on top of a blocked sweat gland. Blisters may form on top of the blocked pore. The whole rash is extremely itchy and made worse by heat and salt in the sea.

Dress the child in cotton clothes keeping hair off the neck. A sun hat will also provide some protection to the chest. Do not over dress or overwrap children who are susceptible. Dry the skin gently after bathing and encourage showers after swims in the sea. Vitamin C found in citrus fruit may help.

HERPES

Herpes simplex is an infection which is caught by contact with someone who is infected. It can be transferred by kissing or during birth if the mother suffers from genital herpes. Children with eczema should be kept away from anyone suffering from herpes. Herpes infection usually is seen around the mouth (see cold sores page 62) with small blisters which ulcerate and

The first infection of herpes is usually mild and requires no treatment. The virus will reappear, however, and the second time it happens the infection is more severe. Antibiotic ointments are available and helpful in this condition, particularly if it becomes infected. The sores usually take about a week to go and are very infectious so keep all washing things separate and wash

CONDITION

spread to the lips. The gums become inflamed and the child will feel generally unwell and may have a fever.

TREATMENT

hands thoroughly after touching the area.

IMPETIGO

Usually occurs after a cold and is an extremely contagious infection. It can spread through scratching to other parts of the body. It is usually first seen around the lips or nose as little blisters which form a yellow scab. If these scabe are picked off the weepy surface underneath is exposed which contains the impetigo bacteria which are transferred and spread. This is when the infection can be transferred to other children.

☆ Treatment should be started as soon as possible
☆ Keep all toilet articles separate and wash separately from the family washing.
☆ Use the ointment prescribed by the doctor and keep the child at home for a couple of days to help prevent the spread of the infection at playgroup or school.

ITCHING — see allergy, athlete's foot, eczema, heat rash, herpes, ringworm, scabies, urticaria

MILIA

Often seen in newborn babies around the face as small white spots. The spots are caused by a blockage of the sebaceous glands in the skin.

No treatment is necessary as they will disappear in a few weeks. Do not squeeze them as they may then become infected.

CONDITION

TREATMENT

MOLES

Small brown marks or swellings which may be hairy or hairless. Moles usually cause no problems but can be removed by surgery if they irritate or embarrass or may cause problems later.

Leave moles alone. If the mole ever becomes larger, more tender or blacker see your doctor. In some cases moles on the soles of the feet are removed because they will be subject to a great deal of pressure once the baby is walking.

MOLLUSCUM CONTAGIOSUM

A round waxy pimple which grows to about 6 mm (¼ in). Over a month or so the pimples may spread. Infection can occur if the pimples are scratched and the condition will spread to the rest of the family if precautions are not taken.

The condition does not have to be treated except that it can spread. It is important to treat children who have any kind of immuno-deficiency or atopic ezcema. Tincture of iodine applied twice daily directly on to the pimple avoiding normal skin will help speed its removal.

MONILIASIS — see Thrush page 71

MOUTH ULCERS

Most ulcers are apthous ulcers though herpes and moniliasis can also cause ulcers. There is no known cause for apthous ulcers though some people seem to be more prone to them than others. The ulcer is small and painful. Ulcers can also be caused

Apthous ulcers need no specific treatment, though the child may be helped by the application of a little teething gel or by sucking an antiseptic tablet. Discourage acid foods such as tomatoes, oranges and vinegar until the ulcer has healed. Frequent

CONDITION

by biting the cheek or tongue. If the ulcer is covered in a white curd-like covering it is likely that it is moniliasis and needs treatment.

TREATMENT

bouts of ulcers can be brought on by stress or an allergy.

MUMPS — see page 46

NAIL INFECTION (Paronychia)

An infection of bacteria or monilia around the nail. It can be caused by an ingrowing nail.

Usually the infection resolves itself in a couple of days. If there is no change see your doctor.

NAPPY RASH

An inflammation of the nappy area caused by a reaction between ammonia and faeces in a dirty nappy. Diarrhoea and allergy to washing powders or fabric conditioner can also cause a nappy rash. Moniliasis is also seen in the nappy area. At first the skin will appear reddened and taut. Later the top layer of skin becomes broken, the skin weeps and becomes ulcerated.

Prevention of nappy rash is by regular cleansing of the baby's bottom at each nappy change. Apply a barrier cream such as zinc and castor oil. If redness occurs, leave the nappy off for a short time at each change and use a cream containing benzalkonium chloride. If the rash is caused by moniliasis or thrush your doctor will prescribe an ointment. Make sure terry nappies are properly sterilized and rinsed and that disposable nappies do not chafe.

CONDITION

TREATMENT

OTITIS EXTERNA

An infection of the skin lining the exterior of the ear which is caused by fungal or bacterial infection. Usually itchy, the skin appears swollen and red and the child may seem deaf. See also page 78.

Make sure ears are dry after bathing and swimming. If there is severe pain and irritation see your doctor for some ointment to clear it up.

PSORIASIS

Seldom seen in children under six years but it tends to run in families. The first attack usually follows a sore throat when red raised spots appear on the skin. After about two weeks they become scaly and disappear. Areas of the body will eventually show signs of the psoriasis particularly knees, back of elbows, chest and scalp. An attack will often occur as a result of stress, or after an injury. Sometimes the nails become pitted.

Psoriasis should be treated by a doctor who will prescribe a suitable ointment. Ultraviolet light is sometimes used and sunlight also helps.

PURPURA

Purple patches in skin caused by bleeding. Often runs in families but can be caused by allergy and reactions to drugs. The lips and gums can also be involved and often nosebleeds occur. Purpura can also cause more severe symptoms of internal bleeding,

If you suspect your child has purpura, see your doctor. Blood tests can be taken to diagnose it and find out the cause.

CONDITION

TREATMENT

inflammation of the kidney and arthritis.

RASH

Rashes are caused by infectious diseases, allergy, heat and can be a sign of general ill-health. If you are unsure of the cause of the rash it is best to speak to your health visitor or doctor.

Rashes occur with allergy, chicken pox, dermatitis, eczema, fifth disease, German measles, heat rash, measles, milia, ringworm, roseola infantum, scabies, scarlet fever and urticaria.

RINGWORM

Caused by a fungal infection of the hair, nails or skin following contact with an infected animal or person. Ringworm can also be caught from pieces of infected hair or scabs. It is found as round flaky patches on the face, arms and scalp. On the scalp it causes bald patches and discolours nails.

Ringworm is treated by an ointment and antibiotics. As the infection can easily be passed on, make sure the child's washing things and bedclothes are kept away from the rest of the family. Any hairbrush or comb used before or during the infection should be thrown away. Keep the child away from school until the antibiotic treatment is complete.

ROSEOLA INFANTUM — see page 55

SCABIES

Scabies is a skin infection that is caused by a minute insect which burrows under the skin to lay its eggs. The eggs hatch and the mites continue to tunnel for two

Treating scabies is by first thoroughly bathing the child followed by the application of benzyl benzoate all over the body. A second application is

CONDITION

weeks when they emerge around the hair follicles, mate and the cycle begins again. Scabies is spread by direct contact with an infested person. The usual signs of scabies are of intense scratching and signs of infestation around the toes and fingers, wrists, palms, armpits, waist, nipples and penis. The burrows of the insects look like small red dots with zigzag grey lines marking the burrows.

TREATMENT

made once the first is dry. The next day two more coats should be applied and all the child's bedding and towels should be washed. In case the disease has spread, the whole family should be treated at the same time. If you have a pet, check that it is not infested as dog scabies can be transferred to humans.

SCARLET FEVER — see page 55

SEBORRHOEIC DERMATITIS

A red scaly rash which occurs mainly in babies with an oily skin. It sometimes leads to eczema later on. It is seen as cradle cap where a scaly crust appears on the baby's head, and in the nappy area. It disappears as the baby gets older.

The baby should be washed using plain water and an unperfumed soap. Cradle cap should be treated as quickly as possible before it becomes too crusty. Use oil to soften the scales and leave on if possible overnight. Most of the scales will rub off but any that persist should have a second treatment a few weeks later. Ask your health visitor about shampoos that are also available.

SORE BOTTOM

Commonly caused by *nappy rash* in a baby. Diarrhoea especially

Children may say that they have a sore bottom meaning they

CONDITION

following a tummy upset and some spicy or acid food can also cause the bottom to appear red and sore. Worms should also be thought of as a cause of sore bottoms in children. Masturbation and child sexual abuse will cause redness in the anal and genital area.

TREATMENT

have several different symptoms. If you are worried talk to your doctor or health visitor. In general, teach your child to wash and wipe their bottom well.

STINGS

There are a variety of insects that can inflict a sting. Calm parents will encourage children to try to ignore wasps and bees, but this is easier said than done. Once the child has been stung fear and panic may set in. Anaphylactic shock is when a child reacts to a sting by becoming pale, sweaty and collapsing. The child must be rushed to hospital immediately. Multiple stings may also need hospital attention. Wrap the area affected with wet cloths and take him to hospital.

Try to reassure the child that the pain will get better soon. Spray the area with a special sting spray if you have one or cool using ice or a cold cloth. There is usually some swelling but this should go down within a day or two. Stings in the mouth can lead to difficulty in breathing. Give the child some ice to suck and take him straight to the doctor. If your child reacts badly to stings and bites, it is sensible to have one of the special sprays to hand during the summer. Your doctor may also prescribe some antihistamine tablets.

THRUSH

Thrush (moniliasis) is a fungal infection which occurs in the mouth and in the nappy area. In

Thrush in the mouth is usually treated by drops and in the nappy area by a cream prescribed by

CONDITION

the mouth it appears as white spots on the inside of the cheeks and on the tongue. These milk-like deposits cannot be rubbed off. The mouth and bottom will both be very sore. Adults may also be infected with thrush particularly on the nipple whilst breast-feeding. Thrush also occurs in the vagina.

TREATMENT

your doctor. You can reduce the risk of a recurrence of thrush by thoroughly sterilizing teats and bottles and by making sure that other members of the family are treated at the same time.

URTICARIA

A rash that is caused by an allergy to a food or drugs or to something the child touches. The rash appears as red itchy weals on the body. There may be severe swelling, pain in the joints, difficulty in breathing and swallowing.

If there is trouble with breathing or swallowing ring your doctor immediately, otherwise bathing in cold water and applying calamine should ease some of the itching. Antihistamines may be prescribed if the allergy is severe.

VERUCCA AND WARTS

Warts are caused by a virus which results in a small growth on the skin. Warts are often found as yellowy lumps on the hands or as brown ones on the face. Veruccas are painful warts on the sole of the feet.

If possible treat the wart as soon as you detect it as they are very infectious. Verucca socks are important if your child swims and in the home make sure that he does not go about barefooted. If the wart or verucca does not disappear with treatment available from the pharmacist, consult your doctor.

Chapter 8

THE EARS AND ASSOCIATED PROBLEMS

Ear infections are one of the most common causes of a visit to the doctor in the first year of a baby's life. Our ears are necessary not only for hearing but also for our balance. The opening of each ear leads to the ear drum and is protected by wax. The other side of the drum is the middle ear which is connected by the eustachian tube which leads to the back of the throat. The inner ear contains the sensitive structures which are concerned with hearing and balance.

The ear acts like a microphone receiving sound waves and converting them into messages to send to the brain. Problem symptoms might include:

Deafness
Dizziness
Discharge
Earache
Excess wax production
Itching or ear pulling

Problems can occur in all three parts of the ear. Some you may be able to see such as a boil, foreign body or excess wax, but others that occur in the middle or inner ear cannot be seen until the child seems unwell. The most common cause of earache is middle ear infection which often occurs with colds and flu, sore throats,

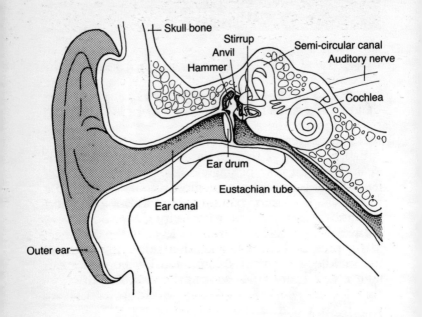

infectious diseases and respiratory infections. If there is a bacterial infection pus forms and presses on the ear drum causing intense pain. If the pain and infection is not treated the drum will eventually perforate and the pus discharge will leak from the ear.

How to give ear drops
Lay the child down on a firm surface with the ear to be treated facing you. Put in the required number of drops and wait a minute or two. Repeat with the other side. It is unwise to use cotton wool to stop the drops coming out as it may get wedged in or pulled out and eaten by the child. Throw away the bottle after the course is completed.

DEAFNESS

Normal hearing depends on soundwaves passing down the ear canal to make the eardrum vibrate moving the three tiny bones in the middle ear. The vibrations are changed to electrical impulses which are carried to the brain by the cranial nerve and are interpreted as sound by the brain. Any damage, disease or malfunction of these structures can cause deafness.

Babies can be born with a degree of hearing loss or deafness, but it is surprisingly difficult to detect in small babies unless special audiological cradles are available in the hospital. Many babies are not found to be deaf until about six months when the baby's sounds in babble will be different from others of the same age. The earlier the baby with a hearing problem is detected the more he can be helped, so if you are worried about your baby's hearing ask your health visitor or GP.

SIGNS TO BE SUSPICIOUS OF HEARING LOSS

☆ Baby does not turn to sounds by 3 months.
☆ Seems startled by your appearance at the cot.
☆ Babbling sounds strange.
☆ Baby not saying a few words by 1 year.
☆ German measles in the mother whilst pregnant.

Only one or two in every hundred deaf children have no hearing at all and so expert help is needed to help him make sense of the sounds that he can hear. It must be remembered that even slight degrees of deafness can interfere with a child's ability to hear speech and can therefore affect language development. Older children can become temporarily deaf after a middle ear infection or even after a heavy cold with catarrh. Check your child's hearing if you are worried.

The treatment for deafness depends on the cause and most forms need specialist help. Antibiotics will cure bacterial infections and drops will remove wax. Glue ear can be improved by the insertion of grommets or drainage tubes. In cases of diagnosed deafness a hearing aid and special teaching can do a great deal to help.

AN A–Z OF CONDITIONS ASSOCIATED WITH THE EARS

CONDITION

TREATMENT

ALLERGY

Repeated ear infections may be a sign of allergy. See page 58.

DIZZINESS

The most common cause of dizziness in a child is an ear infection or an injury to the ear. If possible, it is important to find out what the child means when he complains of dizziness, he may also mean faint, nauseated, or a visual disturbance. True dizziness can be caused by Ménière's syndrome which generally cures itself, but can be worrying while it lasts. Try to observe if there is any loss of balance or jerking movements of the eye. If dizziness persists see your doctor.

Bacterial infection can be treated by antibiotics. Remember to complete the full course.

CONDITION

TREATMENT

EARACHE

Usually caused by a middle ear infection, but it can be caused by mumps, toothache, glue ear, boils and jaw problems.

Warmth helps to ease the pain in an older child. Paracetamol liquid can be given for pain. Call the doctor if the pain persists.

ENCEPHALITIS

An inflammation of the brain caused by an infection. There may be unsteadiness which may be related to an ear infection. The other symptoms are fever, headache, nausea and vomiting, strange movement, neck stiffness and incontinence.

Call the doctor immediately particularly if the child becomes confused or comatose. The child will need to go to hospital for investigation and treatment.

GLUE EAR

Glue ear is a very common form of hearing loss seen in many children under 8 years. It is caused by a sticky fluid gathering in the middle ear. This means that the conduction of sound is impaired with resulting loss of hearing. Glue ear can cause earache, hearing loss and speech problems.

Specialist audiological opinion is usually needed to diagnose glue ear. The child may be given antibiotics or decongestant medicines and nose drops. Sometimes an operation to insert grommets is performed to allow the fluid to drain. Children with grommets need to wear earplugs and a swimming cap if they go to a swimming pool as infection and irritation can occur because of the chlorine in the water.

CONDITION	TREATMENT

MASTOIDITIS

A rare infection these days. It is caused by an inflammation of the mastoid bone and sinuses which has spread from a middle ear infection that has been left untreated. If left without antibiotics it can spread to the brain. The child will have symptoms of otitis media together with redness, tenderness and swelling behind the ear.

The child needs to be seen by a doctor for penicillin injections. The fluid may be drained away by a small operation. Remember to complete any course of antibiotics that are prescribed.

OTITIS EXTERNA

An infection of the skin of the outer ear caused by fungi, bacteria or virus. The child will complain of pain especially on movement and the inside of the ear is itchy and swollen. Check that nothing has been pushed into the ear by the child but do not try to remove it yourself.

An antibiotic medicine or cream may be prescribed. Prevent it recurring by drying the outside of the ear gently after swimming etc. *Never* poke anything inside the ear.

OTITIS MEDIA

Otitis media is a common cause of earache which can only be diagnosed by looking inside the ear. It usually follows a cold, flu, tonsillitis or measles and is caused by a blockage in the Eustachian tubes causing pressure to build up. The child will be in severe

Decongestant nose drops are often given to try to prevent infection of the middle ear. Antibiotics are given together with pain killers for the earache. It can take several months for the child's hearing to return to normal. It is a good idea to have

CONDITION

pain and may have a temperature, loss of appetite and vomiting. In severe cases the ear drum will perforate and there will be a discharge.

TREATMENT

the child's hearing tested about a month after the infection has been treated.

WATER IN THE EARS

Water from the bath or swimming pool can often remain in the ears causing partial deafness. Although it is irritating, it will do no harm unless there is already an infection.

Encourage the child to lie on the side that is affected to allow the water to drain out.

Chapter 9

THE EYES AND ASSOCIATED PROBLEMS

The eyes of a baby or child are often a good indicator of illness. Many feverish conditions are accompanied by sore, red and often sticky eyes, and eyes that lack their usual sparkle may well be telling you that all is not well.

After birth the newborn baby may have swollen puffy or red eyes which result from pressure during labour. This will disappear after a few days but should it recur mention it to your midwife or doctor. A yellowish crusty discharge is also sometimes seen and is commonly known as sticky eye. Your doctor will give you some drops to clear it up. All babies squint during the first few weeks, this is partly due to the folds of skin at the inner corners of the eye which give them a squinty appearance. It takes time for the eye muscles to strengthen but if your baby still appears to be squinting by six months he should be seen by the doctor as early treatment is essential. Most babies cry without tears for about the first six weeks or until the tear glands mature.

Newborn babies have a fixed focal length of about 20 cm (8 in). Quite quickly they will follow a moving face that is close to them and as they grow older their focus will improve. If you are concerned about your baby's vision speak to your health visitor or doctor.

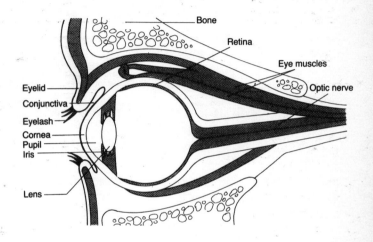

Labels: Bone, Retina, Eye muscles, Optic nerve, Eyelid, Conjunctiva, Eyelash, Cornea, Pupil, Iris, Lens

CHECK-UPS

Your child's vision will be checked by your health visitor or doctor at 6 weeks, 8 months, 15–18 months and on school entry.

HOW TO INSTIL EYE DROPS

Eye drops are usually prescribed for minor eye infections but are difficult to apply because of the blink reflex. Ointment is far easier so if your doctor gives you a choice, opt for the ointment.

1. Wash your hands
2 Lay the child across your lap or on a bed
3. Draw up the right amount in the dropper
4. Put your left arm round the head so that it is cradled and use your finger and thumb to gently hold the eyelids apart
5. Drop in the drops into the corner of the eye just as the eye blinks
6. Allow a few seconds before doing the other eye
7. Wash your hands

The child may complain of a nasty taste in his mouth some minutes later. This is because some of the drops drain down into the throat.

HOW TO PUT OINTMENT IN THE EYE

PRECAUTIONS

☆ Never use one set of eye drops or ointment for another child as eye infections are highly contagious.
☆ Throw away unused portions of eye drops as they have a very short shelf life once opened.

1. Hold the child in the same cradled position as above
2. Squeeze out the required amount onto the inner corner of the eye

3. Keep the child still for a few minutes so the ointment can spread across the surface of the eye
4. Repeat with the other eye. If the ointment does not go into the eye, repeat the application
5. Wash your hands

AN A–Z OF COMMON EYE CONDITIONS

CONDITION

TREATMENT

BLINDNESS

Very few children are born blind, though some are diagnosed at birth with severe cataracts or brain tumours. Blindness may be suspected at about six weeks if the baby does not start to fix its gaze on objects. Toxoplasmosis, toxocara from animals and severe infections can cause blindness. If a squint is not treated the lazy eye will eventually become blind.

If you suspect that your child may have visual problems, talk to your health visitor or doctor. You know your child best so persevere if you are still concerned until you are referred to a specialist. There are large numbers of partially sighted children in Britain, many of whom are able to attend ordinary schools. If a child is completely blind then it may be best for him to be educated in a special school for the blind where his needs will be properly catered for. See Royal National Institute for the Blind (page 125).

BLINKING

This condition is usually noticed when a child is worried about something. It can be caused by itchiness from allergy or conjunctivitis.

Talk to your child about the blinking, he may be able to stop it himself. If there is an emotional cause talking about it will also help.

CONDITION

TREATMENT

BLOCKED TEAR DUCT

The eyes become watery as the secretions do not drain away as normal from the corner of the eye into the nose.

Most blocked ducts clear themselves. If the problem does not go away or there is redness and swelling see your doctor.

CATARACT

A cataract can sometimes be seen as a whiteness of the pupil in the eye. Smaller cataracts can only be seen using optical instruments. They are caused by a variety of different conditions including disease of the mother whilst pregnant (eg German measles). Cataracts can also develop after an injury to the eye or inflammation after an infection.

Usually cataracts are operated on quite early in life. The opaque lens is removed and the baby will wear contact lenses or glasses.

COLOUR BLINDNESS

Most commonly seen as a difficulty to discriminate betwen reds and greens. It is twenty times more common in boys than in girls and hopefully will be detected early so that the child is aware of it.

There is no cure for colour blindness. Children learn to cope in other ways by disinguishing shades. Can be a problem in certain jobs (eg pilot) later in life.

CONJUNCTIVITIS — see Sticky Eye page 80

FOREIGN BODY IN THE EYE — see page 29

CONDITION	TREATMENT

HEADACHES

Headaches can be caused by eye strain but this is rare.

If you suspect that your child has problems with vision get his eyes checked.

LONG SIGHT

An inability to see near objects clearly caused by weak refractive power of lens or cornea, or because the eyeball is too short. The child will screw up his eyes to see nearby objects, have sore eyes from rubbing them and be a reluctant reader.

Long sight should be identified at one of the developmental check–ups. If you are worried ask for a referral to an optician.

MIGRAINE

A severe headache usually on one side of the head. May be accompanied by nausea and vomiting and problems with sight. Migraine is rare in young children. The child may describe flashing lights, a floating feeling or patterns in front of the eyes.

Keep the child in a quiet darkened room. Paracetamol can be given if the child is not vomiting. Migraine can be caused by food allergy.

NYSTAGMUS

Seen as a regular flicking of the eyes from side to side which is not controlled by the child.

The child should be seen by a doctor. It is usually associated with poor vision.

SHORT SIGHT

The child is unable to focus on far away objects but can see near

The child should be seen by the orthoptist so that his vision can

CONDITION

objects well. The condition is usually inherited but may not show up until the child goes to school. The eye ball in these children is too long and the refractive power of the cornea and lens too great. The child will be seen to screw up his eyes, tilt his head or look out of the corner in an attempt to see more clearly. He may appear to hold his book too close to his face, be late in recognizing friends as they run to meet him and have difficulty reading the blackboard.

SQUINT

The child is unable to use both eyes together so that they look in different directions at the same time. A squint is normal in small babies. If the squint is left untreated it may lead to blindness in one eye.

STYE

An infection of the sebaceous gland at the bottom of an eyelash which develops into a small boil. At first the eye appears red, sore and swollen. The stye then appears.

TREATMENT

be thoroughly checked and glasses prescribed if necessary. Encourage the child to wear the glasses as much as possible but not to wear them for close reading of a book. Short sightedness often gets worse at puberty.

If your baby is still squinting by six months, he should be referred to an orthoptist who will thoroughly check his vision. An operation may be needed if treatment with an eye patch does not work.

A hot clean flannel held near the eye will soothe the pain and encourage the infection to come to a head. Boil the flannel after use as styes are very infectious. The stye will burst removing the infected matter from the eye. If it does not burst speak to your health visitor who may remove the eyelash with tweezers.

Chapter 10

THE DIGESTIVE TRACT AND ASSOCIATED PROBLEMS

The process of digestion begins when food is put into the mouth and chewed up by the teeth whilst being moistened by saliva. The food is passed down into the stomach where it is churned around until it becomes a thick mass. Gastric juices start to break the food down so that the digestion and absorption of nutrients can take place further down in the intestines. Rhythmic movements pass the food into the duodenum where bile made by the pancreas breaks down the fats in the food together with protein and carboydrate. The lining of the duodenum allows some of the nutrients in the food to be absorbed straight into the bloodstream. Most of the food passes on into the ileum, where the vilii (small finger-like fronds) remove most of the remaining nutrients. The nutrients are taken in the blood to the liver which is able to convert the nutrients and render harmless any potentially dangerous substances which may have been eaten. The liver also colours the faeces.

In the large intestine water is removed from the food residue making the substance thicker, more carbo-hydrates are absorbed and the residue is bulked up ready for the next bowel movement.

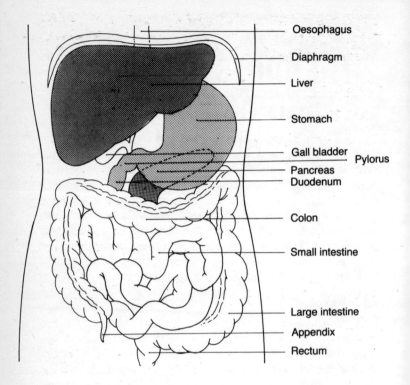

There are several symptoms which may indicate that all is not well with the digestive system. These are:
Diarrhoea or constipation
Nausea and regurgitation
Loss of appetite
Tummy pains and cramps
Jaundice

AN A–Z OF PROBLEMS ASSOCIATED WITH THE DIGESTIVE SYSTEM

CONDITION

TREATMENT

ANAL FISSURE

The child may complain of pain when he goes to the toilet. He may be reluctant to open his bowels and may become constipated. Looking at his bottom you will see soreness and perhaps bleeding around the opening of the back passage.

Increase the amount of fibre (fresh fruit and vegetables) in the child's diet. Offer plenty of drinks too which will help soften the bowel motion and make it easier to pass. A little petroleum jelly may help the soreness too. If the problem persists see your doctor.

ANXIETY

Children may suffer from diarrhoea, constipation or tummy pains if they are very anxious about something. In more severe cases of anxiety the child may have problems eating and may vomit frequently.

Talk to your child to try to find out what has upset him. If you are unable to find out perhaps another trusted adult may be able to help. Occasionally professional help will be needed to help resolve the problem. Talk it over with your doctor or health visitor.

APPENDICITIS

The actual cause of appendicitis is unknown but it is thought to be a result of inflammation produced by food being stuck in the narrow tube or appendix. The

The child needs to be seen by a doctor if you suspect that he may have appendicitis. Do not give him anything to eat or drink in case he needs an operation. A

CONDITION

child will complain of a tummy ache which usually starts near the tummy button and moves out to the right groin area. There may also be vomiting, diarrhoea or constipation and a high temperature.

TREATMENT

diet with plenty of roughage (fibre, ie fresh fruit and vegetables and whole wheat cereals) can help prevent appendicitis.

BAD BREATH

Bad breath can be caused during an illness through a dry mouth such as with tonsillitis, appendicitis or pneumonia. A high fever may give bad breath for a short time. Usually the cause of halitosis is poor tooth cleaning or tooth decay, however some children suffer with it and no cause can be found.

Illness obviously needs treating and hopefully the bad breath will disappear as your child recovers. Check your child's teeth and take him regularly to the dentist. Change the diet to high fibre, low fat and carbohydrate.

BLOOD IN THE BOWEL MOTIONS

Blood can be found in the bowel motion and may appear as red (fresh blood, ie from an anal fissure or piles) or as black when bleeding has occurred higher up the digestive tract.

Look for an anal fissure or piles if you see fresh blood. Ask your doctor if you are worried and also if you suspect that there is bleeding making the bowel motion black. Beetroot and excess blackcurrant juice can also stain the bowel motion especially in babies.

CONDITION

TREATMENT

BLOOD IN VOMIT

Very severe vomiting can result in blood-streaked vomit. If there is bleeding in the stomach the blood will appear black and granular. In breast-fed babies where the mother has a cracked nipple, their dribble or posset may appear bloodstained.

See your doctor if you think your child may have vomited blood. Cracked nipples also may need medical attention if they become infected. Expressing milk is usually sufficient to allow the nipple time to heal.

COELIAC DISEASE

This is a rare condition where the baby is unable to tolerate gluten which is a protein found in wheat, barley, oats and rye. The symptoms usually occur 3–5 months after eating gluten and the child begins to refuse food, loses weight and develops a characteristic pot belly. The stools become offensive.

A diet needs to be advised which is free of all gluten. See your doctor and dietician if you are worried.

COLIC

This is a tummy pain which comes in spasms. Infant colic seems to occur most in the evenings and usually disappears by about 3 months. Both breast- and bottle-fed babies can get colic. Older children may get colic from eating unripe fruit or when they are about to have their bowels open.

Talk to your health visitor if your baby has colic. It is exhausting caring for a colicky baby and you will need advice and support to help you cope. See Cry-sis page 123. Older children will gradually grow through it, but discourage large amounts of fruit if that seems to be the cause.

CONDITION

TREATMENT

CONSTIPATION

Many children will only have their bowels open at home and this can cause constipation particularly if the child will not use the loos at school. Usually however constipation is caused by a low fibre diet, or in some cases an anal fissure which causes pain.

Encourage your child to use the toilet before leaving for school or playgroup. Ask if he wants to go when he arrives at school and if necessary go with him. Increase fibre in the diet by giving more wholegrain cereals, bread and fruit and vegetables. Offer extra drinks particularly of fruit juice. Babies are rarely constipated, and may not need to have their bowels open as frequently as you do! if you are concerned speak to your GP or health visitor.

DEHYDRATION

Dehydration can be very dangerous in a baby and needs to be treated quicly. It can be caused through lack of fluids or through gastroenteritis. Overheating or overwrapping a baby can also cause dehydration. If your child appears listless and unwell especially if it is accompanied by diarrhoea and vomiting get help immediately.

Give extra drinks of water or a rehydration mixture in the case of gastroenteritis. Speak to your doctor if your baby will not take the drinks you offer and is still vomiting. Over-rich feeds can also cause dehydration so read pack instructions on formula milk carefully.

DIABETES

Diabetes is usually caused by an inability of the body to produce

If you are concerned that your child may have diabetes he

CONDITION

enough insulin. This means that the amount of sugar in the blood rises and sugar leaks into the urine. Diabetes may show itself in your child suddenly wanting to drink all the time, loss of weight or in extreme cases a diabetic coma which needs prompt medical attention

TREATMENT

should be taken to your GP to have his blood and urine tested. If diabetes is confirmed he will need daily injections of insulin and careful control of his food intake.

DIARRHOEA

Diarrhoea can be caused by an infection, irritation or allergy to certain chemicals. The child will have his bowels open frequently, often with colicky pains and pass very liquid bowel motions. If the child is otherwise well and has a normal appetite there should be no cause for concern. However, if he seems ill, is vomiting, has tummy pains and no appetite he may need medical treatment.

Offer extra water to drink to prevent dehydration. It may be best to rest the stomach totally for 24 hours and only offer liquids. If the diarrhoea continues seek medical help. Rehydration mixtures are sometimes given.

FAILURE TO THRIVE

A medical term which terrifies parents, but the cause of this can be anything from unhappiness to illness or infection. It does not necessarily mean that you are not a good parent. It is however seen in some cases of child abuse or neglect where the child does not receive enough to eat or has an undiagnosed illness.

As there are many different causes of 'failure to thrive' your GP or health visitor will help to find out the cause and help remedy it. Ask for an explanation if your child is being referred to a paediatrician in these circumstances.

CONDITION

FOOD ALLERGY

A great deal has been talked and written about food allergy and intolerance and parents should be strongly discouraged from restricting a child's diet themselves as it may result in nutritional inadequacy. Before you go to see your health visitor or doctor it may be helpful to make a list of the symptoms that you feel are caused by a food allergy or intolerance.

TREATMENT

Unconventional diagnostic tests such as hair testing or radionics can be unreliable and are usually expensive. A referral to a paediatrician or specialist dietician can aid accurate assessment and the relevance of the symptoms to a dietary cause can be established. If necessary the child can then be put on an elimination diet for a limited period. For useful organizations see pages 122–5.

FOOD POISONING

Food poisoning is caused by infected food which has been contaminated. Salmonella is the most common form of food poisoning. Salmonella poisoning becomes evident between 8–24 hours of eating the food. It is characterised by tummy pains, diarrhoea, vomiting and fever. The illness usually lasts about a week. Staphylococcal poisoning develops more quickly in 2 to 6 hours.

The main danger in food poisoning is dehydration so the child must be given plenty to drink. If drinks are refused, he should be seen by a doctor. A vomiting baby should be seen more quickly, though breast-fed babies are more protected by mother's milk. The prevention of food poisoning is by adequate hygiene in storing and preparing food, and by washing hands after using the toilet.

GASTROENTERITIS

An infection of the intestine often caused by rotavirus which gives sudden diarrhoea, vomiting

As with food poisoning, dehydration is the greatest danger. Plenty of drinks should be given and a

CONDITION

and a raised temperature for up to a week. Rotavirus infection is characterised by a chest infection before the diarrhoea and vomiting.

GINGIVITIS

An inflammation of the gums so that they appear swollen, red and may bleed especially when the teeth are brushed. Gingivitis is usually caused by poor mouth hygiene, mumps, herpes or malnourishment.

HERNIA

A hernia is caused by a weakness of a muscle either near the umbilicus or in the groin which allows part of the gut to protrude abnormally. Usually the hernia feels soft and can gently be pushed back, popping out again immediately. It is not usually painful. A hydrocoele which is a collection of fluid in the scrotum is also sometimes seen with a hernia in the groin.

INDIGESTION

A pain often felt after eating a meal too quickly or too large in size! Occasionally it can be caused by eating something that disagrees with the child.

TREATMENT

light meal if the child feels like it. If you are worried call the doctor, particularly with young babies.

Supervise toothbrushing to make sure that the teeth are cleaned properly to remove the plaque. Anti-bacterial mouthwashes may help in mumps and herpes. See the dentist if the condition continues.

Treatment of hernias is by operation, though it may not be done immediately. If the hernia becomes sore, blue or swollen you should see the doctor immediately as complications may have started which need an operation quickly.

An antacid can help relieve the burning feeling. The indigestion should go of its own accord within a few hours. If you are worried speak to the doctor.

CONDITION

TREATMENT

INTESTINAL OBSTRUCTION

The child may have a swollen tummy and may vomit dark brown or green fluid. There is not usually any pain. It is caused by an obstruction in the intestine which stops the food passing along.

The child needs to be seen by a doctor as an operation may be necessary.

JAUNDICE

In babies jaundice is caused by the immature liver's inability to cope immediately. Other conditions such as abnormalities of the thyroid, the bile system or internal bleeding and infection can also cause jaundice. The skin and the whites of the eyes will appear yellow.

Jaundice in babies is usually treated in hospital by extra fluids and exposure to light. If you are worried that your child has become jaundiced see your doctor.

LEAD POISONING

Lead poisoning is caused by eating or chewing paint, certain cosmetics or inhaling petrol fumes over a long period of time. The child will complain of tummy pains and constipation and may be anaemic with a poor appetite. Unreasonable behaviour is also a symptom and in severe cases, convulsions or coma.

The child needs to be seen by a doctor so that the lead can be safely removed from the body. Prevention is by using lead-free paints especially on nursery furniture and keeping make-up, especially surma, away from children.

CONDITION

TREATMENT

LOW BLOOD SUGAR

Low blood sugar is sometimes seen in new babies. The commonest cause in older children is an inability to maintain blood sugar levels usually after the child has been ill or not had enough to eat. Some children who eat a lot of refined carbohydrate (ie white sugar) may have swings in temperament. Other symptoms include paleness, sweating, yawning, headaches and lack of concentration.

The treatment for new babies will be carried out in hospital until the blood sugar has stabilized. Children with low blood sugars may need a change of diet. Talk to your health visitor or doctor.

MALABSORPTION

Malabsorption is often caused by gastroenteritis but it is also seen in cystic fibrosis and coeliac disease. The child may have a swollen tummy and very smelly bowel motions which are large and pale. After a while poor weight gain and muscle wasting may be seen.

The child should be seen by a paedriatrician to find out the cause of the problem. Often the cause is simply a bad bout of gastroenteritis from which the child has not recovered. Cutting down on milk and sugar will encourage the lining of the intestine to repair itself but this should be done with care to make sure that the child remains properly fed.

MILK INTOLERANCE

Only 7% of babies and children are really milk intolerant. The symptoms are those of a tummy

The treatment of babies and children with suspected cow's milk allergy or intolerance should

CONDITION

upset, skin problems, respiratory upset and failure to gain weight.

TREATMENT

always be with the guidance of your doctor or health visitor. This is particularly important for bottle-fed babies.

OVERWEIGHT CHILDREN

Some children do seem to have an inborn tendency to put on weight easily. The most common cause is still too much food particularly of the wrong sort. Fat children are more likely to to become ill and they may suffer emotional and physical problems.

The child's diet must be looked at in relation to the rest of the family. Is he allowed to eat sweets in between meals, what does he eat at school? Talk to the school nurse who may well be able to encourage healthy eating. Regular exercise by the whole family will also help.

PROLAPSED RECTUM

This can happen after severe constipation when the child has had to strain hard to go to the toilet. You will be able to see part of the rectum protruding and the child may complain of a lump in his bottom.

The prolapse can be treated at home by laying the child down and raising the foot of a sofa or bed. Some toilet paper or kitchen roll should be wrapped round your index finger and the rectum pushed gently back inside. Do not remove the paper — it will come out with the next bowel movement. Tell your doctor if it happens again. Prolapse can be prevented by giving a high fibre diet with plenty of drinks.

CONDITION

TREATMENT

PYLORIC STENOSIS

If your baby suddenly starts vomiting two to three weeks after birth and becomes constipated, pyloric stenosis may be suspected. The vomit usually shoots out of the mouth. The baby will cry for food and yet vomits immediately. It is caused by a narrowing of the stomach's outlet into the small intestine.

If you suspect that your baby has pyloric stenosis ask your health visitor to come and watch a feed. Your doctor will then refer the baby for an operation to relax the tight muscle, though in some cases medicine may be enough.

RICKETS

Rickets is caused by a lack of Vitamin D. It may be lacking in both the diet and the child's exposure to sunlight. Bone deformities at the rib cage and spine together with knock knees and bow legs are common signs. There may also be constipation, irritability and tooth decay.

Extra playtime in the fresh air unencumbered by too many clothes will increase the body supply of Vitamin D. Vitamin drops may well be advised but Vitamin D is found naturally in eggs, butter, cheese, liver, tinned fish and cod liver oil.

SICKNESS — see Vomiting page 101

SUGAR INTOLERANCE

Sugar intolerance can occur after gastroenteritis but if it occurs after 3 years it is often a true sugar intolerance which is particularly seen in black or Chinese children. The child will complain of tummy pains, a sore bottom and some diarrhoea.

Cutting down on milk may well relieve the symptoms though this should be done under medical guidance as milk is a vital part of a child's diet. Cut down on other sugary foods too and see if the symptoms improve.

TONGUE FURRING

A slight whitish furring on the tongue is normal but if the child is ill the furring may become thick and offensive. Thrush is also seen as white furry patches but this needs medical treatment.

Keep the child's mouth clean by regular toothbrushing and mouthwashes if he is ill. Offer plenty of drinks.

TOOTHACHE

The child may be reluctant to eat and the symptoms of pain and earache may be made worse by hot or cold food.

Paracetamol suspension may temporarily ease the pain, but the child needs to be seen by a dentist.

TRAVEL SICKNESS

Travel sickness is actually thought to be caused by an imbalance in the middle ear. It usually is seen in children over the age of 6 months peaking before 10 years and disappearing by adolescence. Signs of imminent travel sickness are sudden silence, sleepiness and paleness. Sweating, tears and mouth watering mean that the child may soon vomit. Keep an old ice cream container in a plastic bag in the car so that you are well prepared.

Train travel seldom causes travel sickness and is therefore worth considering where possible. The front seat of the car is often preferable for children who are travel sick providing they are correctly fastened into a seat belt. Many children are less sick if they travel in the afternnon or evening. Do not give a child a full meal before travel. Offer snacks such as crisps, barley sugar or dry biscuits and avoid fizzy drinks. Cold water is best and causes no problem if spilt! Tablets can be prescribed for travel sickness though they can have unpleasant side effects.

TUMMY ACHE

Many children complain of tummy pains and these can be of either physical or emotional symptoms. Infections such as mumps and measles, indigestion, allergies and diabetes and asthma can also cause tummy pains. There may be other symptoms which will give an indication of what is wrong, such as diarrhoea, vomiting or a sore throat.

Emotional problems often express themselves as tummy pains as it is the child's way of gaining attention. Try to find time to talk alone to find out the cause of it.

When a child is in pain, try to find out as much as possible about it before you give a pain killer such as paracetamol suspension. Find out how long it has been going on, whether it is in the same place all the time and whether anything strange has been swallowed by accident! If the pain continues, contact your doctor particularly if the child becomes lethargic or you are worried.

VOMITING

Vomiting can happen because of many infections or illnesses in children. If there is blood (red or black) you will need to take your child to the doctor.

Offer sips of drink and later a little toast if the child is hungry, gradually increasing food and drinks if there is no further vomiting. If you are worried contact your doctor particularly if he becomes irritable or very drowsy suddenly or if the vomiting occurs after a fall or blow to the head.

WORMS

Threadworms, round worms, whipworms, hook worms and tape worms are all able to live in

If you suspect that your child has worms see your doctor. You may need to provide a specimen of

the human body. Threadworms which are the most common cause itching around the bottom and soreness of the vagina in girls. It is particularly noticable at night. Other worms may cause tummy aches, diarrhoea, wheezing and actual damage to organs of the body. See also Chapter 12.

the child's bowel motion for laboratory analysis. Usually worm killing medicines are prescribed. Make sure that the whole family are treated if necessary and clear and refresh bedding and all surfaces in bedrooms after treatment. Take special care if you have cats and dogs as pets and ensure they are regularly wormed.

Chapter 11

RESPIRATORY INFECTIONS

Breathing is a bodily function we do not need to think about until something goes wrong. Chest infections, sore throats, asthma, coughs and bronchitis are some of the most common childhood ailments and can be extremely worrying to parents as the most difficult moments often occur at night.

The lungs do not function before birth and so the first indication of how well they are going to work is the first cry that a baby makes. With this first breath the lungs inflate and fill with air and the oxygen passes into the baby's circulation rather than via the placenta and umbilical cord which has carried the oxygen to the baby in the womb. The adult respiration or breathing rate is 12–20 breaths each minute. Children's rate is 20–30 and a baby breathes about forty times each minute.

The respiratory system defends itself against infection by a very active lining which excretes fluid which contains antibodies to infection. Large particles of dust become trapped in the hairs which line the upper part of the respiratory tract and become embedded in the mucus until the nose is blown and they are removed.

There are several symptoms which may indicate that all is not well with the respiratory system. These are:

High temperature
Sneezing

Coughing
Mouth breathing
Discharge from the nose
Phlegm from the throat
Nosebleed
Wheezing
Hoarseness

As children become more sociable and join playgroups, mother and toddler clubs and so on, they become vulnerable to a multitude of infections. The prompt recognition of symptoms can often help prevent a cough or cold turning into a more severe infection not only in your own child but also amongst other children. Some children may be more vulnerable to chest infections for instance if they are asthmatic or have cystic fibrosis.

HOW TO GIVE NOSE DROPS

Lay the child down on a firm surface and put his head slightly to one side and tilted back so that the drops do not run straight out. Put in the required number of drops, wait a minute or two and then repeat on the other side. The child may well complain of a nasty taste as the drops may go down the back of the throat. Throw away the bottle after the course is completed.

AN A–Z OF ILLNESSES ASSOCIATED WITH THE RESPIRATORY SYSTEM

CONDITION

TREATMENT

ALLERGY

See asthma and hayfever

If the child becomes wheezy, has a runny nose, cough, rash or tummy ache it may be a response to something he is allergic to. This only happens in about 1 in 5 children and such children need specialist help to identify and thereby avoid the allergen.

ASTHMA

Asthma is an allergic condition which causes a narrowing of the air passages and an outpouring of the mucus which makes the child wheeze and find breathing difficult. Dust, grass pollen, animals and foods are all common causes of asthma, but emotional stress can also trigger an attack.

Asthma attacks usually occur at night with the child waking up unable to breathe out. Panic sets in and help is needed urgently. Asthma affects about 1 in 20 children and seems to affect more boys than girls. Many children grow out of it in the

Call the doctor if this is the first attack your child has had. Sit the child up and try to calm him by putting on a record or tape or reading a favourite story. As he relaxes more air will be allowed through into the lungs.

The doctor will prescribe drugs which can be given at the start of an attack but if the attack is already underway an injection may be the quickest way to relieve the symptoms. Try to find out what has caused the attack and remove the allergen if possible.

Physiotherapy to help the child learn to breathe correctly is

CONDITION

teenage years, but whilst they have it, it can put a great deal of stress on the family who care for them.

TREATMENT

helpful and antibiotics may be given at the first sign of any cold or cough to help prevent an attack. See page 122 for further information.

BLUE SKIN

Many babies have blue fingers and toes even when they are warm and tucked up. This is nothing to worry about and is caused by the lack of maturity of the blood vessels in their hands and feet. Some congenital heart defects are the cause of blueness of the skin because there is not enough oxygen circulating in the blood.

All 'babies are examined by a doctor before they leave hospital to check for heart defects. If you are worried about your baby, speak to your health visitor or doctor.

BREATH HOLDING

Breath holding looks very alarming especially to a parent, but it is not dangerous. It usually occurs in older babies in the middle of a tantrum or whilst screaming. It occasionally may lead to a convulsion. Once the baby has held his breath long enough to become unconscious, a reflex causes breathing to start.

Try to remain calm as the more attention the child gets, the more likely he is to repeat breath holding. Talk to your doctor or health visitor if it gets to be a problem every time you say NO!

CONDITION

TREATMENT

BRONCHIOLITIS

This is an infection of the smallest air passages which is mostly seen in babies under six months particularly in winter and spring. The baby may wheeze, cough and go blue and the baby may need to be cared for in hospital. Often the baby has been in contact with children or adults with respiratory infections and it is for this reason that it is best not to allow too much kissing of small babies.

Call the doctor if you suspect that your baby may have bronchiolitis. Prop the baby up so that it is easier for him to breathe until the doctor arrives.

BRONCHITIS

An infection which causes inflammation of the lining of the bronchial tubes. It is often caused by viruses so antibiotics are not often given. Wheezing and coughing are common especially in overweight children. The British climate is often blamed for the amount of bronchitis in this country, but it is also commonly seen with infections of the sinuses, tonsillitis, cystic fibrosis and congenital heart disease. The child usually has a cold for a few days and then starts to cough and feel short of breath. Later the cough becomes productive and phlegm is made which can cause vomiting.

Cough medicine and antibiotics do not usually help. Encouraging the child to spit up phlegm helps as does physiotherapy to the chest. Place the child's head down over the knees of a seated adult and pat the back vigorously.

CONDITION

TREATMENT

CATARRH

Catarrh is an increase in the normal amount of mucus in the nose, throat, ears and sinuses. Many children are sick after swallowing a lot of catarrh particularly at night. The child may also appear slightly deaf and may have diarrhoea.

Catarrh can be caused by infected polyps and adenoids which may need removing. The doctor may prescribe decongestants if the symptoms are very severe though this can eventually be counter-productive. It usually disappears after a few days.

CHAPPED LIPS

Dry, sore lips which may bleed can be caused by a severe respiratory infection or fever. It is made worse if the child licks his lips.

The lips need protection by using a barrier cream such as zinc and castor oil cream or petroleum jelly.

COLDS

Colds are caused by viruses which attack the lining of the nose, throat, sinuses and ears. Most children have colds regularly through the year once they go to playgroup or mix with others. Colds are not caused by severe chilling though this may lower a child's resistance. Colds in babies can seem alarming with a runny nose, sore throat and sneezing. Babies become restless but rarely have a high temperature. In older babies the first sign of a cold may be a

Keep your child at home if he has a temperature or is very infectious and sneezing all the time. Teach him to blow his nose by holding one nostril closed with a finger and blowing down the other. Protect the skin under the nose with a barrier cream. Offer the child plenty to drink and if breast-fed feed him more frequently. If the cold seems to be turning to a chest infection see the doctor, otherwise it is not necessary unless you are worried. A little eucalyp-

CONDITION

fever. Occasionally nose drops are prescribed to allow a baby to feed more easily.

TREATMENT

tus oil sprinkled on to the night clothes at bedtime will help the child breathe more easily.

COUGH

Anything that irritates the throat or airways can cause a cough as it is a reflex reaction which we are all born with to clear mucus that might otherwise impair our breathing. Usually coughs are caused by an excess of mucus caused by a cold, but they can also be caused by asthma, bronchitis, whooping cough and pneumonia, so if in doubt see your doctor.

Cough mixtures that suppress the cough should only be used at night if sleep is being badly disturbed. Antibiotics are of little use as coughs are usually caused by viruses. Encourage the child to cough up phlegm as it may otherwise lead to diarrhoea and vomiting.

CROUP

Croup is a form of laryngitis which can affect babies dramatically as their breathing tubes are so small. The child usually wakes with croup at night, with a loud, hacking cough which causes them to cry as it is painful. On taking another breath you will hear a barking/crowing noise which sounds most alarming. He will hardly be able to speak. If you think the child is finding it hard to breathe and his lower chest is sucked in with each breath call a doctor urgently.

Try to calm the child as the more he panics the less oxygen he will be able to take in. Open a window and encourage him to take some deep breaths as the cold moist air will help reduce the swelling inside the larynx. Then run a bath or shower or boil a kettle (safely) in the room to make the air humid. Keep the child in the room for 10 minutes or until the doctor arrives. If your doctor cannot come quickly call an ambulance or take the child to the nearest casualty de-

CONDITION

If your child has a tendency to croup it is worthwhile buying a vaporiser from the chemist and using it at night if he has a cold or cough.

TREATMENT

partment. If the croup is caused by a bacterial infection, antibiotics may be prescribed and anti-allergy medicines if it is caused by an allergen.

CYSTIC FIBROSIS

Cystic fibrosis is an inherited disease which produces an excess of sticky mucus in the lungs, pancreas, sweat glands and bowel. One in 2000 children has the disease which is often discovered at birth as an obstruction of the intestines. Later it can cause respiratory infections, failure to gain adequate weight, constipation or diarrhoea and prolapse of the rectum. The paediatrician will test for cystic fibrosis using a sweat test and the earlier it is detected the better the outlook for the child.

Treatment is by special diet and added enzyme medicine. Antibiotics, inhalations and physiotherapy for chest infections. For further information and support see page 123.

FLU

Flu or influenza is a viral infection of the upper respiratory tract. It is a highly contagious infection which occurs in epidemics and is transmitted by droplets from nose and throat discharges of people who have the disease. It has a short incubation period of 1–3 days and is contagious for

Keep the child in bed whilst he is feeling weak and aching. Call the doctor if you suspect that he has an ear infection, sinus problems or a severe chest infection as antibiotics may be needed. Offer plenty to drink to bring down the temperature and replace the fluids lost by sweating.

CONDITION

seven days before the symptoms occur. It appears first as a cold and sore throat followed by sweating and high temperature, painful limbs and back, coughing, vomiting and diarrhoea.

HAYFEVER

Hayfever is an allergic reaction of the membranes of the nose and sinuses to inhaled substances. It can be caused by seasonal factors such as pollen of trees or grasses, or be perennial due to cats, dogs and cows. Feathers, house dust and moulds can also cause hayfever.

The child will have a discharging, inflamed nose with redness, itching and watery eyes. There is often a headache. The symptoms last for as long as the allergen is around. If the child has allergic inflammation he may be more vulnerable to bacterial infection.

HICCUPS

Hiccups are caused by a spasmodic contraction of the diaphragm which causes the short sharp noise we call a hiccup. Babies have been seen to hiccup on ultrasound scans long before they are born.

TREATMENT

Try to isolate the cause of the hayfever and keep the child away from it if at all possible.

Medicines are given by doctors to help the allergic rhinitis and decongestant nose drops and antihistamines can be useful during a prolonged attack.

Hiccups in children are seldom serious. If they last for more than a day, speak to your doctor. Otherwise try out one of the popular remedies — occasionally they do work! Make the child hold his breath for a count of 10 or breathe into a paper bag.

| **CONDITION** | **TREATMENT** |

HOARSENESS

Hoarseness can be caused by croup, allergy, laryngitis or by straining the voice. Always check that there is not a blockage in the throat. In severe cases the voice is lost completely.

Keep the child's throat warm by wrapping a scarf around the neck. Give plenty of warm drinks and if possible use a humidifier which moistens the air. The child should be seen by a doctor if you suspect that the hoarseness is caused by an allergy.

LARYNGITIS

Usually caused by a viral infection during the winter. The larynx becomes inflamed and later infection of the trachea, lung or middle ear may occur. Laryngitis frequently follows a severe cold or flu and is sometimes caught after one of the childhood infections. Laryngitis in babies is a rare but serious condition needing medical help. The symptoms include hoarseness, sore throat, a dry cough and croup.

The child will breathe more easily if the air is humidified (preferably with cool rather than hot vapour). If necesary antibiotics may be given to treat a suspected bacterial infection. If your child seems to have difficulty in breathing get medical help immediately.

PLEURISY

Pleurisy is an inflammation of the lining around the lung which allows fluid to accumulate making it difficult for the child to breathe. It occurs occasionally with pneumonia and certain types of cancer. The child will complain

Your doctor should be called so that treatment can begin quickly. It is sometimes necessary for the child to be treated in hospital. Antibiotics may be given.

CONDITION

of chest pain which is worse when he strains or coughs. The pain is often felt in the back or the shoulder. The child may breathe more quickly than usual, grunting and appearing rather blue around the lips.

TREATMENT

PNEUMONIA

An infection of one or more areas of the lungs caused by bacteria or a virus. Pneumonia can also be caused by an allergy, irritant fumes, vomit or an inhaled foreign body. The symptoms include a mild respiratory tract infection followed by a sudden high fever. The child will feel cold and cough in short rapid breaths. There may be chest pain and some children have a stiff neck and tummy pains.

The child needs to be seen by the doctor so that treatment can be given quickly. Bacterial pneumonia will respond well to antibiotics providing the full course is given. Occasionally a child may have to go into hospital.

SINUSITIS

An inflammation or infection of the sinuses. Because the sinuses are part of the nasal cavity they can be affected by any viral infection or allergic reaction of the nose. The symptoms include a high fever, pain, stuffy nose and a cough. Depending where the infection is sited there may be headaches or swollen eyelids.

Antibiotics may be needed if there is a bacterial infection. Otherwise paracetamol suspension can be given for pain. Decongestant nose drops will help the child to feel he can breathe more easily.

CONDITION

There will be a yellow/green discharge from the nose.

SORE THROAT

It is often hard to detect a sore throat in babies and toddlers, but a reluctance to eat or swallow may indicate the cause of the problem. The child may complain of tummy pains and earache. Sore throats are often accompanied by a cold, infection of the ears or sinuses and swollen glands.

TONSILLITIS

The tonsils' function is to destroy disease-causing germs. They may become mildly or chronically infected with these germs and appear enlarged, red and in some cases infected. In most cases the glands in the neck will be swollen and painful.

TREATMENT

Offer plenty to drink though the child may be reluctant to swallow. Straws may help as will ice cream. Doctors vary as to whether antibiotics are necessary, but if they are given, make sure that the course is completed. Paracetamol can be given for pain and some children find a gargle helps.

The treatment is the same as that for a sore throat. Tonsillectomy is not done as frequently as it was in the past as children often grow out of the frequent sore throats by the time they are seven or eight. Check your child's hearing following a severe case of tonsillitis.

Chapter 12

WORMS, HEADLICE AND OTHER NASTIES!

Most parents feel not only a little squeamish but also guilty and ashamed if they are told that their child has one of the nasties! One of the main problems with all infestations is that because the public do not feel at ease talking about them they become a taboo subject not only for the parents but also for the children. The only way to stop the continual round of headlice treatment and worm infestation is to tell people that your child has been in contact with, once it has been diagnosed, and advise them of the appropriate action.

Many schools and playgroups send home slips of paper or letters to inform parents that there are headlice in the class, but because of the reluctance of parents to admit to worms it is still a common problem at school. If you are fed up with treating your child perhaps you could raise the subject for discussion at the next PTA meeting. If you feel too shy, you could speak to the child's teacher or school nurse, failing that you could write to the head having asked a couple of friends to support you.

THREADWORMS

Threadworms are the most common worm infestation in Britain. It has been estimated that as many as 40% of children under 10 years are affected by this persistent visitor. A smaller but significant number of parents also play host to this unwelcome guest. Threadworms are more of a nuisance than a disease. They can be treated but are likely to recur unless the whole family is treated at the same time and strict hygienic measures are taken whilst the condition is present.

Threadworm eggs are commonly passed from child to child by hand contact. The eggs will be present under the nails of the infested child and can enter the host's body by hand to mouth or hand to nose contact. The eggs hatch under the stimulation of the digestive juices, and the immature worms live for about 14 days feeding in the intestine. Mating then takes place and the male dies. The female worm travels down to the rectum and waits until the child is warm in bed, then wriggles through the anus and lays her eggs. The eggs are sticky and cling to the creases of the anus. The wriggling causes irritation which leads to the child scratching and the transfer of eggs to the fingers and nails ready for the cycle to begin again. The cycle takes four to six weeks to complete and so a treatment is often prescribed that can be repeated 14 days after the first dose thus killing any more females that have come to maturity.

The intense itching is the only clear symptom which is apparent. It becomes worse at night and can cause sleep disturbance and subsequent irritability. Bed wetting occurs in some children and others complain of tummy pains. The worms can make their way into the urinary tract of girls and produce symptoms of a urine infection. Treatment is available from your doctor in the form of tablets or powder. Some preparations are

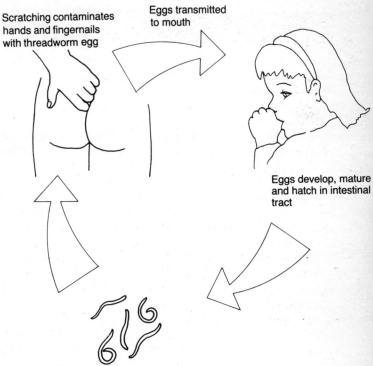

Scratching contaminates hands and fingernails with threadworm egg

Eggs transmitted to mouth

Eggs develop, mature and hatch in intestinal tract

Adult worms emerge from the anus at night and lay eggs on the surrounding skin

available from your pharmacist. Do not forget to buy enough for the whole family and start the treatment at the same time. It is not advisable for these drugs to be taken in the first three months of pregnancy.

Drugs alone will not eliminate threadworm infestation. Where possible the children should wear pyjamas in bed or a nightie with pants. The bed sheets should be changed after treatment and the bedroom and bathroom dusted and vacuumed thoroughly. The eggs can survive for several days in dust and infected garments. The fingernails should be kept short and particular attention should be paid to handwashing after going to the lavatory and before meals. A bath or bottom wash in the morning will remove any eggs laid during the night.

Do not forget to tell the school or playgroup so that reinfestation can be prevented.

ROUNDWORMS AND WHIPWORMS

These worms survive where sanitation is poor or where human sewage is used as a fertiliser. With the increase in foreign travel, about a thousand cases are diagnosed annually in Britain. Diagnosis is made by laboratory examination of the faeces as in the case of children they are often symptomless.

The adult worm is about 30 cm (12 in) long and lives in the small intestine of the host. About 200,000 eggs are evacuated daily with the faeces and it is here that contamination of vegetables can occur if it is used as manure and the produce is not washed.

The most common complication of infestation is intestinal obstruction which usually will respond to drug treatment before surgery is needed. Roundworms can be treated by the same powder as is used for threadworms.

The roundworm toxocara canis which can infect dogs and cats can infect children by contact with the infested animal faeces. These pass into the child's gut and can eventually cause blindness and epilepsy. For this reason it is essential that house pets are regularly wormed. If your animal has a skin infection or is scratching excessively take it to the vet to be treated. It is not advisable to allow your children to kiss animals or let the animal 'kiss' the child. Keep feeding bowls separate and do not let your pet eat from the family's dishes.

TAPEWORM

Tapeworm infestation occurs mainly as a result of eating undercooked pork. In most cases the first sign of infestation is the presence of flat white segments in the stool. Until the head of the worm has been removed the segments will continue growing and so careful examination of the faeces needs to be carried out once treatment has started.

HEADLICE

Headlice are extremely common amongst school children today and are increasingly seen on pre–school children at playgroups and mother and toddler groups. As with worm infestations, the only way to eradicate lice is by treatment of all contacts and the close family. The family may well include grandparents too! Even if you do not see grandparents very often it may be that they may reinfest your child at every visit, so do not forget to ask them to check their own heads! Headlice prefer clean hair but are happy to move to any head with short or long, clean or dirty hair. They are spread by direct head to head contact with someone who already has headlice. It usually takes 4–6 weeks for the new host to discover that he has headlice.

So what should you look for? An itchy scalp is often the first sign that a child has headlice, if the child is seen scratching especially around the ears, take a look. The headlouse is a small brown/grey insect which lives close to the scalp. The eggs are known as nits which are firmly attached to the hair and cannot be shaken off or brushed off. The cast-off skins may be seen when combing a child's wet hair. Another sign of headlice

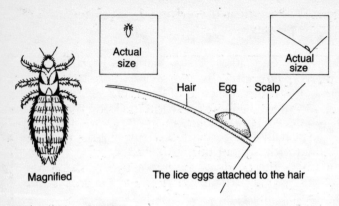

Actual size

Actual size

Hair   Egg   Scalp

Magnified

The lice eggs attached to the hair

How to recognize headlice.

infestation is the presence of brownish powder dust on the pillow in the morning. This is the droppings from the adult headlice. If you find that your child has headlice, ask your school nurse, health visitor or pharmacist which lotion is most appropriate. Headlice become resistant to these lotions so you must check to see that you use the most effective one.

Headlice shampoo is not very effective though it is easier to use. The lotion is usually more successful providing it is used as follows:

1. Apply the lotion to the *whole* scalp.
2. Allow it to dry naturally — do not use a hairdryer. Leave at least 2 hours but overnight is best.
3. Wash the hair as usual.
4. Treat all the family, but take care with children under 1 year.
5. If your child suffers from eczema or asthma ask for a water-based lotion.
6. There is no need to comb out the treated nits unless you want to — they will not live or lay eggs.

Once you have treated everyone the next thing to think about is prevention.

PRECAUTIONS

☆ Make sure each member of the family has his or her own comb and brush and uses it daily, especially before bed. Combing injures the lice and makes them unable to lay eggs.

☆ Check the heads of the family before shampooing, paying particular attention to the crown and behind the ears.

☆ If you are regular swimmers, remember that chlorine makes the lotion less effective. Try to leave the lotion on overnight as this will prevent reinfection for longer.

SCABIES

Scabies is a skin infection which is caused by the mite sarcoptes scabei, a crawling insect which is barely visible. See page 69.

USEFUL ORGANISATIONS

Action on Smoking and Health (ASH)
5–11 Mortimer Street
London W1N 7RH
(071–637 9843)

Alcohol Concern
305 Gray's Inn Road
London WC1X 8QF
(071–833 3471)

Association for Post-Natal Illness
7 Gowan Avenue
London SW6 6RH
(071–731 4867)

Association for Spina Bifida and Hydrocephalus
22 Woburn Place
London WC1H 0EP
(071–388 1382)

Asthma Society
300 Upper Street
Islington
London N1 2XX
(071–226 2260)

British Diabetic Association
10 Queen Anne Street
London W1M 0BD
(071–323 1531)

British Homoeopathic Association
27a Devonshire Street
London W1N 1RJ
(071–935 2163)

Child Accident Prevention Trust
28 Portland Place
London W1N 4DE
(071–636 2545)

Child Growth Foundation
2 Mayfield Avenue
London W4 1PW
Information on normal growth rate of babies and young children particularly those with lack of growth hormone.

Child Poverty Action Group
4th floor, 1–5 Bath Street
London EC1V 9PY
(071–253 3406)

Children's Legal Centre
20 Compton Terrace
London N1 2UN
(071–359 6251)

**Cleft Lip and Palate
  Association (CLAPA)**
Hospital for Sick Children
Great Ormond Street
London WC1N 3JH
  (071–405 9200 ext. 5289)

Community Health Councils
Address and phone number of
  your local Community Health
  Council in your local
  directory. Advice, where and
  how to get the service

**Contact a Family with a
  Handicapped Child**
16 Strutton Ground
London SW1P 2HP
  (071–222 3969)

**Council for Complementary
  and Alternative Medicine**
19a Cavendish Square
London W1M 9AD
  (071–409 1440)

Cry-sis
BM Cry-sis
London WC1N 3XX
  (071–404 5011)

**Cystic Fibrosis Research
  Trust**
5 Blyth Road
Bromley
Kent BR1 3RS

**Down's Syndrome
  Association**
12/13 Clapham Common
South Side
London SW4 7AA
  (071–720 0008)

Gingerbread
35 Wellington Street
London WC2E 7BN
  (071–240 0953)

Haemophilia Society
123 Westminster Bridge Road
London SE1 7HR
  (071–928 2020)

**Hyperactive Children's
  Support Group**
71 Whyke Lane
Chichester
West Sussex
  (0903 725182)

**Institute for Complementary
  Medicine**
21 Portland Place
London W1N 3AF
  (071–636 9543)

Maternity Alliance
15 Britannia Street
London WC1X 9JP
  (071–837 1265)

**Meet-a-mum Association
  (MAMA)**
3 Woodside Avenue
London SE25 5DW
  (081–654 3137)

Mencap (The Royal Society for
  Mentally Handicapped
  Children and Adults)
123 Golden Lane
London EC1Y 0RT
  (071–253 9433)

National Association for Mental Health (MIND)
22 Harley Street
London W1N 2ED
  (071–637 0741)

National Caesarean Support Association
72 Perry Rise
London SE23 3QL

National Childbirth Trust
Alexandra House
Oldham Terrace
London W3 6HN
  (081–992 8637)

National Childminding Association
8 Masons Hill
Bromley
Kent BR2 9EY

National Council for One Parent Families
255 Kentish Town Road
London NW5 2LX
  (071–267 1361)

National Deaf Children's Society
45 Hereford Road
London W2 5AH
  (071–229 9272–4)

National Eczema Society
Tavistock House North
Tavistock Square
London WC1H 9SR
  (071–388 4097)

National Information for Parents of Prematures: Education, Resources and Support (NIPPERS)
49 Allison Road
Acton
London W3 6HZ
  (081–992 9310)

National Marriage Guidance Council
Herbert Gray College
Little Church Street
Rugby CV21 3AP
  (0788 73241)

NSPCC
67 Saffron Hill
London EC1N 8RS
  (071–242 1626)

National Toy Libraries Association
68 Churchway
London NW1 1LT
  (071–387 9592)

NAWCH (The National Association for the Welfare of Children in Hospital)
Argyle House
29–31 Euston Road
London NW1 2SD
  (071–833 2041)

One-Parent Families
225 Kentish Town Road
London NW5 2LX
  (071–267 1361)

Parents Anonymous
9 Manor Gardens
London N7 6LA
(071–263 8918)

Pre-School Playgroups Association
61–63 Kings Cross Road
London WC1X 9LL
(071–833 0991)

Royal National Institute for the Blind
224 Great Portland Street
London W1N 6AA
(071–388 1266)

Sickle Cell Society
Green Lodge
Barretts Green Road
Park Royal
London NW10 7AP
(081–961 7795)

Spastics Society
12 Park Crescent
London W1N 4EO
(071–636 5020)

Standing Conference on Drug Abuse (SCODA)
1–4 Hatton Place
Hatton Garden
London EC1N 8ND
(071–430 2341)

Thalassaemia Society United Kingdom
107 Nightingale Lane
London N8 7QY
(081–348 0437)

Twins and Multiple Births Association
c/o Mrs Jenny Smith
41 Fortuna Way
Aylesby Park
Grimsby
South Humberside DN37 9SJ

Vegan Society
33–35 George Street
Oxford OX1 2AY
(0865 722166)

Vegetarian Society of the UK
Parkdale
Dunham Road
Altrincham
Cheshire WA14 4QG

Women's Aid Federation
(England)
52–54 Featherstone Street
London EC1Y 8RT
(071–251 6537)

Women's Health and Reproductive Rights Information Centre
52 Featherstone Street
London EC1Y 8RT
(071–251 6580/6332)

Working Mothers Association
23 Webbs Road
London SW11 6RU
(071–228 3757)

SUPPORT AND HELP IF YOU LOSE YOUR BABY OR CHILD

Compassionate Friends
6 Denmark Street
Bristol BS1 5DQ
  (0272 292778)

Foundation for the study of Infant Deaths (Cot Death Research and Support)
15 Belgrave Square
London SW1X 8PS
  (071–235 1721/0965)

Miscarriage Association
18 Stoneybrook Close
West Bretton
Wakefield
West Yorkshire
  (0924 85515)

Stillbirth and Neonatal Death Society (SANDS)
28 Portland Place
London W1N 3DE
  (071–436 5881)

Support After Termination for Abnormality (SATFA)
29–30 Soho Square
London W1V 6JB
  (071–439 6124)

INDEX